Disability Bioethics

Series Editors: Hilde Lindemann, Sara Ruddick, and Margaret
Urban Walker

*feminist
constructions*

Feminist Constructions publishes books that send feminist
ethics in promising new directions. Continuing the work of
feminist ethics critique, it emphasizes construction, aiming to build a positive body of
theory that extends feminist moral understandings.

Disability Bioethics
Moral Bodies, Moral Difference

Jackie Leach Scully

ROWMAN & LITTLEFIELD PUBLISHERS, INC.
Lanham • *Boulder* • *New York* • *Toronto* • *Plymouth, UK*

ROWMAN & LITTLEFIELD PUBLISHERS, INC.

Published in the United States of America
by Rowman & Littlefield Publishers, Inc.
A wholly owned subsidiary of The Rowman & Littlefield Publishing Group, Inc.
4501 Forbes Boulevard, Suite 200, Lanham, Maryland 20706
www.rowmanlittlefield.com

Estover Road
Plymouth PL6 7PY
United Kingdom

British Library Cataloguing in Publication Information Available

Library of Congress Cataloging-in-Publication Data:

Scully, Jackie Leach.
  Disability bioethics : moral bodies, moral difference / Jackie Leach Scully.
    p. ; cm. — (Feminist constructions)
  ISBN-13: 978-0-7425-5122-0 (cloth : alk. paper)
  ISBN-10: 0-7425-5122-9 (cloth : alk. paper)
  eISBN-13: 978-0-7425-6457-2
  eISBN-10: 0-7425-6457-6
  1. Disabilities—Moral and ethical aspects. 2. Disabilities—Social aspects. 3.
Medical ethics. 4. Bioethics. I. Title. II. Series.
  [DNLM: 1. Disabled Persons. 2. Bioethical Issues. 3. Eugenics. 4. Feminism. 5.
Moral Obligations. 6. Reproduction—ethics. HV 1568 S437d 2008]
  HV1568.S388 2008
  179'.7—dc22   2008012825

Printed in the United States of America

⊗™ The paper used in this publication meets the minimum requirements of
American National Standard for Information Sciences—Permanence of Paper
for Printed Library Materials, ANSI/NISO Z39.48-1992.

Contents

Acknowledgments

This book owes debts to many people. My attitudes to disability were shaped by my mother, Lilian Emily Scully, and later at Cambridge University by Margaret Spufford and Derrick Puffett. Tom Shakespeare was one of the first to encourage my academic interest in disability, although he would probably want me to point out he has disagreed with me a lot ever since. Christoph Rehmann-Sutter listened to my grumbling about bioethics' treatment of disability, and guided my early research questions. He has also made many insightful comments on the manuscript. Rouven Porz's questions about virtually every point I make have also helped clarify my thinking.

I've been greatly helped over the years by the thoughtful responses and respectful dissent of colleagues in bioethics and disability studies. These colleagues are too numerous to list by name but I particularly want to express my gratitude to the members of the Swiss Society for Biomedical Ethics, and to the Feminist Approaches to Bioethics Network, which continues to be exceptionally supportive of disability issues within bioethics. My thanks also to colleagues in sociology and in the Policy, Ethics and Life Sciences Research Centre at Newcastle University, and especially to Stephanie Lawler for her comments on chapter 6. Grateful thanks also to participants in the courses on disability I have run at Woodbrooke Quaker Study Centre, Birmingham, UK, and to the Disability Equality Group of Britain Yearly Meeting.

Some of the ideas in the book were tentatively floated at a National Endowment for the Humanities summer seminar on *Justice, Equality and the Problem of Disability*, held at Sarah Lawrence College, New York, in summer 2002. All the participants left some imprint on my thinking, but Vrinda Dalmiya, Debora Diniz, Christian Perring, and Sophia Wong are among those most likely to recognize the outlines of our conversations, as would Rosemary Quigley, if she were still with us. I'd like to thank the leaders of that seminar, Eva Feder Kittay and Anita Silvers, for their continued encouragement and support.

Parts of the material, especially from chapters 4 to 6, have been presented in a variety of forms and locations, including at the Disability Studies Association, Lancaster, in 2004, and the 2004 Feminist Approaches to Bioethics Network Congress, in Sydney; workshops at Macquarie University and Wollongong University, New South Wales, in January 2006; and lectures at the European Molecular Biology Laboratory, Heidelberg, in 2005 and at the Albert-Ludwigs-Universität, Freiburg, in 2007.

Special thanks to Alison Peacock for a conversation at Rheinfelden that encouraged me to pursue the idea; Andrew Lovett, for ever-probing questions at a distance; Astrid Pfründer, for making clear my limitations; Trevor Jackson, for an unwittingly helpful comment about the case of Ashley; and Marta Buckland, for houseroom in summer 2007. And it would be remiss of me not to acknowledge here the technical support, first provided by audiologists of the National Health Service, later by Hörberatung Schwob, Basel, and most recently by the UK's Access to Work scheme, which makes my working life possible.

Monica Buckland Hofstetter not only talked the talk and walked the walk, but read the draft, checked the proof, prepared the index, made the tea, and generally held the fort. All this while attending to her own vocation. A righteous muso, indeed.

1

Bioethics and Embodied Difference

> How is it possible that nondisabled people tend to feel sorry for me? It
> still takes me by surprise. . . . The widespread assumption that disability
> means suffering feeds a fear of difference and a social order that doesn't
> know what to do with us if it can't make us fit its idea of normal.
>
> —Harriet McBryde Johnson

In autumn 2005, a statue appeared on the unoccupied fourth plinth in London's Trafalgar Square. The piece, by Marc Quinn, depicted a nude woman,
and in this it was not exactly unusual in the history of art. However, it was
anomalous in several other respects. The first was that it was a public piece,
and the commemoration of a woman in public art is rare, let alone in such
a prestigious and symbolically significant site. The second was that the
woman was eight months pregnant, and outside of defined contexts, such
as medical television programs, the public depiction of pregnancy, especially naked pregnancy, makes many people uneasy. And finally, the figure
had vestigial arms and legs. The model, a woman named Alison Lapper, was
born with a condition known as phocomelia.

Alison Lapper: Pregnant created quite a stir, in a muted English way. Not
because she was a woman in a space traditionally reserved for military he-
roes, nor because of the very visible pregnancy, though those issues came
into it. The real problem was what was *not* there: normal arms and legs. It
became clear that many people had difficulty accepting an impaired body
as suitable for public view. Discussion of the statue's artistic merits in the
end took second place to a debate about disability and its meaning in contemporary British society. Among the things these discussions revealed
were that disability becomes very complex when it interlocks with gender

and social status; that many people are dismayed at the idea of disabled people having children; that we are not sure if a person should be valued *because of* or *in spite of* or *irrespective of* an impairment; and that a lot of assumptions are made about the relationship between physical variation, impairment, and quality of life. At the time, several people remarked to me that Lapper's impairments were tragic but that luckily, medicine could now "do something" about it.

It's the task of bioethics to consider the morality of what medicine can *do about* things. In this book I argue that bioethics has an interest in disability that goes deeper than questions of regulating reproductive choices, its prime focus so far. There are biomedical technologies today that can be used to prevent the birth of people with genetic or congenital impairments, and many people think the use of these technologies must be regulated; bioethicists have already had a lot to say in this context. Beyond that, it may not seem that there is much else about disability that is ethically interesting. We all know, or think we know, what disability is. (Although the lines here are more contested than they appear.) We all know, or think we know, that having an impairment is not something anyone would want. (Although the choices made by some people call this into question.) And we also agree, or at least pay lip service to the agreement, that however undesirable it may be to have an impairment, disabled people themselves have political and civil rights, including rights of access to and participation in civil society. So not much to argue about ethically there, perhaps.

There are other reasons why bioethicists might just not feel drawn to spend their time thinking, talking, or writing about disability, unless they have their own vested interest in it. Most of us find the notion of a failing or defective body emotionally difficult, especially when the body is our own. Thinking about bodily impairment, illness, or trauma is upsetting, and we will—at least consciously—avoid doing it if we can. Even the available vocabulary seems to make it harder rather than easier to talk about impairment. The word *disability* is unavoidably negative. Structurally it signifies a loss or a lack, a state that exists only because it falls short of something better. It's worth noting, too, that the word we use is *dis*-abled, not *un*-abled. The prefix *dis* points to something taken away or displaced: it refers to the way someone ought to have been, rather than how he or she is now. The word *disabled* also homogenizes whatever it splits off. *Disabled* never specifies exactly what it is I am unable to do. It's as if there is no need to, because the details of what I cannot do are not nearly as important as the simple fact that I can't. To be disabled, in our language and culture, means to be identified as globally incompetent (Fuss 1989, 4).

Yet the unfriendliness of this cultural and linguistic environment belies the fact that over the last twenty years or so, the conceptualization of disability has altered dramatically. Advances in biology, and major political and social changes, are opening up a space in which physical and mental deviations from the norm mean something more complicated and interesting than a straightforward story of individual bad luck. Disability today can be conceptually framed as an emancipatory movement and minority rights issue; a biomedical phenomenon; an emergent political identity; a set of social relationships and practices; and, most recently, a field of legitimate academic inquiry. Disability studies looks beyond (but, in my opinion, should not exclude) the biomedical understanding of impairment and toward its cultural representations and social organization. In shifting emphasis like this, disability studies marks itself off from medical sociology, which has stayed closer to the deficit/repair paradigm and which has concentrated more on acute and chronic illness than on disability (Thomas 2007). The emergence of disability studies has made it possible to study impairment as one form of variation among humans, without feeling either pity for the subjects of inquiry or apologetic for having such a perverted interest. In this way, disability joins the general late twentieth-century trend of attending to *difference* as a "significant and central axis of subjectivity and social life" (Corker 1999, 630). Similar paths from obscurity to academic respectability have been taken by related studies of otherness such as women's and gender studies, black studies, queer studies, and so on—although the parallels between disability and these other emancipatory-movements-turned-academic-domains break down at some important and theoretically revealing points. But one thing they do have in common is that they are not just "about" particular marginalized identities. As well as expanding our knowledge of impairment and its consequences, taking disability into consideration "adds a critical dimension to thinking about issues such as autonomy, competence, wholeness, independence/dependence, health, physical appearance, aesthetics, community and notions of progress and perfection—issues that pervade every aspect" of our lives (Linton 1998, 118), and all of them issues with which bioethics constantly grapples.

For those of us whose personal and professional lives have been influenced by the changing face of disability, things are now both simpler and trickier. Simpler, because if we want to, we can choose to collapse the multiplicity of ways in which it is possible for the human body to be anatomically and physiologically variant into a single *sociopolitical* concept of disablement. (Not all of us find this collapse either helpful or empirically accurate, though.) Trickier, because to speak of disability *ontologically*, as a way of being, rather than *pathologically, as a way of being medically out of whack*, is to replace a well-charted set of questions with less-familiar ones. If disability is a way of being, what sort of being is it? How exactly does it develop? Which (that is, whose) representations of disability have authority? What relationship does disability have to other social or ontological categories, like gender, ethnicity, or class? Is disability in fact a genuine ontological category—is it really an authentic way of being, or is it just a useful organizing category for a motley collection of odd bodies? And if it *is* an identity, can it ever be anything other than a spoiled one (Goffman 1971) that we are morally obliged to restore to normality if we can, or prevent happening if we can't?

Ironically, disability's migration from pathology to ontology has taken place just at the point when it has become normal to turn to biomedicine for authoritative answers to the questions of human existence. In the half century since a structure for deoxyribonucleic acid (DNA) was published, and since restriction enzymes made the controlled micromanipulation of DNA feasible, the science of molecular biology has hugely enlarged our understanding of living organisms. It has also helped transform our expectations of medicine and is beginning to change actual medical practices. As a result, medical ethics and bioethics today are dominated by the need to deal with the questions thrown up—sometimes, it feels, on a daily basis—by advances in molecular genetics and reproductive science.

Even a casual observer of these medical ethical and bioethical discussions notices how they tend to repeat well-trodden lines of argument. One of the most popular and powerful rhetorical devices used to back up medical intervention is the therapeutic imperative. What, after all, "could be controversial about the goal of improving human life through the application of a scientific knowledge of genes?" (Buchanan et al. 2000, 264). Since contemporary society has a strong drive to medicalize—to describe features of life in biological terms wherever possible, so that their problematic aspects become things best dealt with biomedically—to say that something is therapeutic now trumps virtually all other considerations. When it comes to impairment, the absolute priority of the therapeutic imperative as a general principle has been questioned by some bioethicists on the grounds of distributive justice, healthcare economics, or even of overall benefit to the patient. What bioethics has signally failed to address is the cluster of prior and crucial questions about the *ontological* and *moral character* of bodily variation. Can this form of embodiment be considered an identity, a way of being? Can it be a *desirable* way of being? This possibility entails questions about when and how variation becomes impairment or disabling, and why it matters. And given the choice, would and should we prefer a more normal way of being?

It seems obvious that the difficult task of setting ethical limits to medical intervention in disability is not made any easier if we still disagree about fundamental questions of what impairment or disability actually is. We need to remember, though, that the question of disability's ontological and moral status has not come up in quite this form before, because fretting about *what ought we to do?* is pointless until something can, realistically, be done. And until recently, all that biomedicine could do about disability was to intervene in the lives of existing disabled people through treatment, amelioration, or rehabilitation.[1] While genetic knowledge has long been used to *minimize* the transmission of unwanted characteristics from one generation to the next, today's technologies—and some that are widely anticipated for the future—offer radically new options for *preventing* it. Now it is one thing to have an *opinion* on disability; opinions take on quite different significance when they are the grounds for concrete, effective actions, particularly when those actions include preventing the existence of certain kinds of people. This is why it has become urgent to take a close look at those opinions, identify where they come from, and evaluate the extent to which they are ethically justifiable.

THEORIZING THE DISABLED BODY

Fortunately for those of us interested in exploring disabled embodiment, the body has recently become intellectually fashionable in disciplines other than medicine. This multi- and transdisciplinary engagement places bodies within a number of conceptual frameworks. Bodies can be tackled biologically or medically, phenomenologically, through their material or social relations, as discursive constructions, as psychically established through internal representations, and so on. Most scholars agree that any one of these approaches in isolation can provide no more than a partial account of a phenomenon as complex as embodiment, and furthermore that the traditional dualisms of mind and body, or culture and nature, probably will not generate the most faithful accounts of the ways bodies come to inhabit the world.

Within an appealing conceptual diversity, however, two frameworks currently dominate academic thinking about the body. Representing opposite ends of a disciplinary spectrum, neither has adequately grasped the ethical significance of embodiment, and each of them has its own difficulty in finding a theoretical space for statistically unusual embodiments. At one extreme is biological, or these days usually genetic, reductionism, which seeks purely biological explanations for human characteristics and behavior. Genetic reductionism uses the popular but oversimplified picture of gene action in which DNA sequences (molecular biologists call this the genotype) encode instructions for proteins that ultimately determine people's bodily characteristics (or phenotype), from their hair color to their sexual preferences, and especially their health. According to this model, genes provide the most fundamental (and therefore, in reductionist terms, the best) account of human embodiment.

It is important to emphasize here that not all of genetics is reductionist, and that reductionism is often analytically and methodologically appropriate in biology. Still, the main problem with genetic reductionism as popularly practiced is its tendency toward essentialism, and the reification of one genotype as species typical. It implies that there is a canonical genotype (or at best, set of genotypes) that contains the blueprint for the normal phenotype, and that any variations from that genotype (and by inference that phenotype) are to a greater or lesser extent abnormal. It does not seem to me that this kind of essentialism in fact follows from molecular biological evidence, and I have argued elsewhere (Scully 2002, 2006a) that there are convincing alternative ways of imagining gene action. The point I want to highlight here is that if genetics is used primarily in a dichotomous way to identify and separate the genotypically normal from the abnormal, it cannot *at the same time* be used for a nuanced investigation into the characteristics of whatever it is separating off as abnormality. It thus encourages the homogenizing of all variance.

It's also worth noting that a genetic approach to embodiment often manages to sidestep the meaty stuff entirely. In a genetic model, the ultimate generator of embodiment is not even the chemical deoxyribonucleic acid but *information*. The genetic code is a heuristic that nevertheless stands in a causal relationship to proteins, cells, tissues, and biological processes. The genotype is certainly closely connected to the phenotype that the organism ends up with, but in a way that involves a disjunction at the point where we reinsert the construct of code back into the biology we are trying to understand. The picture of a conceptually simple and linear path from gene to complex human behaviors also skips over the further disjunction between phenotype and being. Molecular biology is not (yet) in a position to predict a person's health and behavior with reasonable certainty from genetic information alone, nor to say much about what that person's life will be like. Its power to provide *descriptions* of the human body in terms of constituent genes and cellular processes, though, leads very readily to assuming that the level of genes and cells is also an appropriate place to find an account of living *with* or *as* or *in* a particular kind of body. This is an important distinction to keep in mind: since ethics is about living and not chemistry, it is surely accounts of lived experience, and not biomedical description, that should form the basis for morally evaluating types of embodiment.

At the other extreme from genetic reductionism lie diverse poststructuralist and postmodernist strands of contemporary thought, celebrating plurality, challenging the naturalization of identities and norms, and understanding the self as constructed in the course of social interactions that inscribe identities on bodies. These approaches all recognize that the biological body never presents to us *as is*, in a presocial, unmediated form. Any grasp we have of it is always from a particular historical, cultural, and political viewpoint. It might be intriguing to imagine what a completely unsocialized human would make of the body, but barring methodologically and ethically questionable experiments, we can do no more than imagine it. Moreover, as embodied humans investigating embodiment, we are in the thick of things: we can't remove ourselves to some detached point from which we can reflect on what being bodied means. None of these statements is particularly radical nowadays, and a postmodernist approach provides important criticism of normalized representations of bodies. But the discursive turn becomes problematic when the idea that there is a biological substrate to embodiment slides out of sight entirely. There is then nothing to stop theory from becoming untethered from materiality, forgetting that bodies have real constraints (including anatomical and biochemical ones) that limit their redescription or transformation. The metaphor of the body as a *surface* of inscription also neglects what happens on either side of the surface, that is, the body's own intrasubjective and intersubjective capacities.

A postmodern nonjudgmental celebration of plurality can also be as effective a device for avoiding anomalous embodiment as any more obviously normalizing discourse. The postmodern rejection of the grand narrative of normality and the decentering of the normal subject are both ways of shifting our conceptual framework so that we no longer feel obliged to think of *variation* as *deviation* from a norm. Yet doing so can also remove much of the basis and rationale for making analytically useful comparisons. If the postmodern challenge to norms, including bodily norms, also manages the feat of "disappearing" the normative physical body, it effectively removes the possibility of being able to *notice* the difference that is there. For example, the claims by some disability advocates that "anyone can be disabled" or even that "everyone is disabled because nobody is perfect" can be seen as important attempts to undermine the normal/abnormal dichotomy. But it can also mean that the real difficulties that exist are dismissed before they are properly addressed. As the late Mairian Corker noted with some asperity, "Those who emphasize the fact that everyone can become disabled while ignoring the fact that not everyone is, are denying disabled people's reality—in fact they abandon the notion of reality altogether" (Corker 1998a).

Neither biologically reductionist nor postmodern approaches have enough to offer as resources for understanding variant bodies ontologically or morally. Indeed, it seems intrinsically unlikely that any one theory of the body could give an adequate account of the diversity of disabled embodiment. To the intellectual difficulty of comprehensively theorizing any kind of embodiment, disability adds a requirement to account for the complete range of impairments. Even if a unified theory of disability were possible, a different question is whether it would be desirable. And here the postmodernist answer would be that it is not; the thing to do, rather, is to place a

ﾑltiplicity of theoretical frameworks around the problem, accepting that, in the end, they may turn out to be incommensurable. The difficulties that this solution presents for any movement with practical social and political change in mind have been well rehearsed in feminist and postcolonial critiques of postmodernism.

ETHICS AND THE BODY

Ethics has to do with bodies because morality is concerned with behavior, and behavior involves bodies. However abstract ethical theory becomes, and however generalized the rules given in guidelines and legislation, at the heart of theories and rules lie concerns about regulating what embodied actors do to each other. Our capacity for moral concern evolved in social groups where interactions and their consequences were more direct than they often are now. A basic moral sense arises out of the awareness that individuals are vulnerable to each other in their bodily interactions: moral concern would be a very different thing if we were able to float around the world in a disembodied way.[2] But even choices that touch others only indirectly, as is often the case for political or economic decisions, are made by an *embodied* consciousness, and much of this book details how the specifics of body and place are significant for moral understanding as well. Driven by moral concern, then, ethical rules are attempts to prevent or minimize the damage done (and to maximize any benefits) when embodied humans interact.

It is now a well-rehearsed criticism of traditional moral philosophy that it does not take bodies seriously into account in the way this sketch of morality would suggest. When philosophers talk about "moral agents," they are more concerned with agential capacities for rational thought, or with emotional or behavioral characteristics, than with their physical ones. Greek and Judeo-Christian roots have produced a Western philosophical tradition with a preference for envisaging the self as a disembodied locus of consciousness, free to reason in any way since reason is transcendent and not bound by bodies or cultures. Post-Enlightenment ethical thinking also takes as paramount the idea that morality must be universalizable, not just locally generalizable. This has generally been interpreted as meaning that in their morally relevant features people are interchangeable, or ought to be treated as if they were. It has seemed obvious to most philosophers operating within this tradition that questions of the rightness and wrongness of actions, or goodness and badness of character, or what should count as a moral principle or as a virtue, have little to do with *physical* selves. Neither moral psychology nor philosophy has taken bodies as sources of moral insight, and moral philosophy has been prone to see them as rather more of a liability.

The picture of the moral self as a bodiless, rational, atomized decision-maker overlooks significant areas of moral life, like relationships, community, or social history. These are the areas that have always been central to feminist and other heterodox philosophical strands that balance ethics' traditional individualism with a more collectivized viewpoint. The fact that some bioethicists are taking more systematic interest in the social context within which moral decisions are made, and incorporating empirical data as valuable for normative ethical reflection, is a shift in philosophical practice. But with the major exception of feminism's attention to the ethical consequences of bodies being *gendered*, bioethics still does not take adequate account of the differences that result from variations in embodiment.

The claim of this book is that impaired or disabled embodiment is worth closer bioethical attention. What we really think about bodies that differ from the norm is ethically important, because our beliefs about normal embodiment inevitably become normative: they determine what we hold to be the right kinds of bodies to have or be. They also determine the degree of effort to normalize anomalous bodies we think is appropriate. When we draw lines between bodies that are normal and those that aren't, or those that are simply variant and those that are outright impaired, these decisions are normative ones that reflect how we think bodies *should* be, and that indicate how far we are prepared to go to be sure of getting the bodies we want. Later on, I will be arguing that normative ethics involves attending to the construction of our values and desires, trying to understand where they have come from and how they are justified. The challenge of unusual embodiment is that it poses unexpectedly hard questions of justification to the normative ethical reflections that are performed from a nondisabled perspective (that is, most normative ethics). These hard questions, however, are precisely what bioethics needs to ensure that it is properly critical and self-critical when it addresses issues of importance to disabled people.

ETHICS OF DISABILITY/DISABILITY ETHICS

There seem to me to be two fundamentally distinct ways of thinking about disability in ethical terms. One I will call the *ethics of disability*, the other *disability ethics*. The ethics of disability is the systematic reflection on morally correct ways to behave toward disabled people—in everyday interactions, in healthcare or employment policy, or in law. By disability ethics, on the other hand, I refer to the particular moral understandings that are generated through the experience of impairment.

The ethics of disability are necessarily both specific (they are about disability) and general (they must seem reasonable to both disabled and nondisabled people if they are to have any real moral force). Disability theorists have not paid as much attention to the ethics of disability as they could have. Disability studies grew out of political movements in Britain and the United States that were stirred to action by noticing and experiencing injustice. The field now flourishes through its ability to conceptualize topics related to disability as "simultaneously and ontologically both personal and public" (Williams 2001, 123). And it is a young enough discipline for some of its adherents still to feel that it might change the world, a belief that takes an ethical stance toward the world as it is. But largely for reasons of history and disciplinary politics, disability theorists' ethical reflection has been conflated with and overshadowed by a strong political agenda. Even though much of what goes on under the broad heading of disability studies has an implicit ethical commitment derived from its emancipatory goals, the ethical dimension is not often made explicit. The unraveling of what is wrong with a "disabling society" and why it needs changing, for example, works from the premise that all members of society, including its disabled members, have the same rights of access and civil participation. But these are sociological or political analyses that tend not to draw on relevant ethical theories, for example of moral personhood or justice, to back up their claims.

By contrast, mainstream bioethical literature *has* tackled issues that are button-pushers for disability. Bioethicists working within one or more of the frameworks of moral philosophy have shown an interest in the ethics of euthanasia and medical treatment decisions at the end of life, healthcare rationing, prenatal testing (PND), preimplantation genetic diagnosis (PGD), the reproductive choices of disabled people (especially when disabled people want to use reproductive medicine to become parents),[3] or gene therapy. Another difficult area is the use of medicine and biotechnology to normalize variant bodies or minds, which becomes more morally troubling when it involves parental choices about children, as it often does; examples include limb-lengthening surgery for people with restricted growth (Parens 2006), cochlear implantation into infants or very young children, and so on. One high-profile case in early 2007 involved Ashley, a multiply disabled girl whose parents requested hormonal treatment and surgery to make her physically easier to manage, and therefore care for at home, as she reached puberty (Gunther and Diekema 2006; Butler and Beadle 2007; Wilfond 2007).

Most bioethicists take a highly normative approach, not least because bioethics is routinely asked to justify the regulatory frameworks established for biomedicine and biotechnology (skeptics see this as proving bioethics to have much the same legitimizing function for biomedicine as Sinn Fein once had for the provisional IRA). And following the dominant Anglo-American influence in bioethics and medical ethics, the consideration of disability issues has a strongly libertarian and utilitarian flavor. Moreover, and unlike in disability studies, there are few disabled bioethicists and even fewer who take disability as a focus for their work. While some bioethical writing on disability has been sympathetic to disability concerns and has begun to show the imprint of the work coming out of disability studies itself (e.g., Edwards 2004), it is overwhelmingly produced from the standpoint of outsiders to the experience being written about (Harris 1995, 2000; Buchanan 1996; Nelson 2000a; Parens and Asch 2002).

Here are two significant intellectual communities contributing in very different ways to the ethics of disability: mainstream bioethics, in which ethical analysis is the focus but the view is from the outside; and disability studies, where statements are more likely to be made by people who know, experientially, what they are talking about, but where ethics has so far played a supporting role to a predominantly social and political project. Despite the differences in their contributions, both communities are doing what I have defined as the ethics of disability, or thinking systematically about morally proper stances and behavior toward disabled people. It is a central argument of this book that we also need another kind of ethical engagement with disability. Disability ethics, like feminist ethics, is a form of ethical analysis consciously and conscientiously attentive to the experience of being/having a "different" embodiment. Where feminist ethics' concern is with the non-normativity introduced by gendered bodies, however, disability ethics looks at the embodied effects of impairment. And doing this means working from people's experience of disability to see if and how it colors their perceptions, interpretations, and judgments of what is going on in moral issues, especially in moral issues that have direct relevance to disability and where differences in the experience of disability might be expected to have weight.

Understanding how embodiment affects the moral world requires more empirical and more phenomenological approaches than are generally taken by either disability studies or bioethics. Empirical investigation goes some way to providing the kind of data that would indicate whether or not there are relevant differences in disabled people's practices, attitudes, and opinions around bioethical issues. If some or all disabled people make choices, hold opinions, or prioritize particular goods that are different from those of some or all nondisabled people, we could say they have different moral understandings. We would not be claiming that they are utterly different, or even that they differ in the most important respects; we would be claiming only that there are differences worth noticing and that might be ethically relevant. Empirical studies of social, historical, economic, political, cultural, or relational circumstances may then go some way toward providing an explanation for commonalities and divergences.

But while empirical work may illuminate what the features of life as a particular body are like, it makes no attempt to say what it is like to *be* that embodiment. For this we need a more phenomenological approach. Phenomenology recognizes that a subject's sense of self, her perceptions and understandings of the world, are inextricably bound up with her body and its interactions with other bodies and with her environment. A phenomenological take on ethics acknowledges that moral understanding is dependent on how the subject experiences her presence in the world, which from a phenomenological point of view is an accumulation of everyday bodily events and encounters.

Michel Foucault described the work of phenomenologists as "unfolding the entire field of possibilities connected to daily experience," and he didn't mean it as a compliment (Foucault 1991, 31). Phenomenology stands in sharp contrast to the poststructural/postmodernist theorizing of complex human phenomena, like disability, as the products of discourses and networks of domination. Foucauldian poststructuralism's view of the body as object of knowledge and subject of power has been particularly influential in sociology and critical theory, and latterly in disability theory. It has provided a powerful strategy for uncovering the discourses and associated social artifacts and practices through which bodies are culturally legitimized and regulated. Nevertheless, the poststructuralist way has its own problems. I suggested earlier that an exclusive commitment to uncovering discourses carries the epistemological risk of missing the stubbornly prediscursive living body. (Bodies *are* before they speak or are spoken about.) But there is an attendant ethical danger, which is to lose sight of the particular vulnerabilities and strengths of given embodiments. If, as I suggested earlier, it is just these vulnerabilities and strengths that determine how bodies interact harmfully, then ethically responsive societies need to know about them. Otherwise, we will have no data against which to test our assumption that people whose experience of embodiment is *other* will share everyone else's ideas about goods and harms. Without those data our efforts at ethical line-drawing will necessarily be based on extrapolation from a limited set of standard experiences and will inevitably protect the interests of some groups at the expense of others. I say more about the ethical consequences of this in chapters 3 and 8.

Narrative is a particularly powerful way of doing phenomenologically thick accounts of the experience of disability, and in chapter 6 I look at disability narratives as providers of moral identities. One of the distinguishing features of disability is that it most often affects people with no previous experience of it: notwithstanding the current fascination with genetic or congenital impairment, the majority of disabled people acquire their impairment in the course of their postnatal lives, through aging, disease, or trauma. Disabled people generally have to learn how to be disabled, often without anyone around to show us how. Even when impairment is present from birth, many disabled children have little or no contact with anyone who can show them the skills which they will need to survive and flourish. (Such isolation can be an unexpected side effect of efforts at educational mainstreaming, for example.) They have to find out how to cope with the practical demands of their impairment, as well as with any relational changes or effects to their sense of self after the onset of impairment. At whatever stage of life impairment becomes apparent, the person with a physical disability must integrate identity and body function in ways that differ from the common experience, "to accept a variant body image and to learn to use the body automatically and unselfconsciously in culturally acceptable ways" (Frank 1986, 189). Contact with other disabled people or with written disability narratives can be a significant support to this learning process. Memoirs and mentors help structure an epistemology of the disabled experience, which is also a moral epistemology: these accounts are sources of information about how to be a "good" disabled person, and what are the right choices for a disabled person to make—about how to do disability well.

Getting at other ways in which the disabled experience shapes subjectivity is not quite so straightforward. The incorporation of social relationships happens at a level of consciousness, and the preverbal structuring of cognition at a stage of development, that render both transformations almost beyond articulation. Nevertheless I suggest that some way of uncovering and conveying these dimensions of experience is necessary for a fuller understanding of disability ethics. In chapters 4 and 5 I try to do so, first by drawing on the sociologist Pierre Bourdieu's influential theory of the *habitus*, and then by looking at the philosophy of Maurice Merleau-Ponty, relating his phenomenological work to recent studies in cognitive science that connect bodily experience with the semantic and metaphorical structuring of moral thinking.

Critics of a phenomenological or body experiential turn in disability theory raise a number of points of difficulty. One is that it can rely on a naive notion of experience as self-evidently present to us, and epistemologically transparent, when in reality the concept of experience is, as Gadamer encouragingly put it, "one of the most obscure [ideas] that we have" (Gadamer 1986, 310). From Kant onward, philosophers and scientists have been (mostly) agreed that our knowledge of what goes on in the world around us is inevitably mediated. Knowledge does not just happen but is painstakingly acquired through the operations of the senses, cognitive processes, and culture-specific acts of interpretation and evaluation. So we never have access to a person's experiencing of an event or (via that experience) to the event itself: all we really have are accounts (our own and other people's) which are selective and partial, both because constructing any story entails selection, but also because the prior *experiencing* did so as well. Those who have taken the discursive path in contemporary thought would go further and claim that there is simply no such thing as prediscursive experience. It is not that we encounter the world and then put words to the experience so that we can make sense of it to ourselves: experience is just not present to us until structured through language. Experience is "always already an interpretation and something that needs to be interpreted" (Scott 1991, 797). And claims to the incontestable authority of experience render it impossible to examine the assumptions and practices behind it.

Feminists, of course, have been here before. The starting point for feminist theory and methodology is the insistence that women's experiences are different from those of men—different enough, anyway, to make them worth investigating. This stance is still foundational for feminism. Yet it was also from within feminism that the question was asked: Whose experiences get to "stand for" women in general? What are the unexamined political and epistemic choices that are made when we start to speak of a group's experience? These are questions I come back to in chapter 7. Moreover, once we acknowledge the basic impossibility of the phenomenological project to "bracket out" all theoretical presuppositions of what an experience means, then it becomes clear that the articulation of experience can be profoundly conservative. The narrative and cognitive frameworks through which we make sense of our lives are made available through the cultures in which we live, and may be morally damaging. I take this up again in chapter 6.

It is nevertheless possible to acknowledge the limits of what we can know from accounts of other people's experience, and still find them useful in exploring moral worlds. After all, if it is the case that no one has unmediated access to brute reality, then our own moral understandings are constructed around bits and pieces of biased reporting just as much as our attempts to grasp another's. The understandings of everyday life are undeniably fragmented, skewed, often incoherent or even mistaken. We can work within an acknowledgment of these limitations and at the same time avoid falling into an uncritical use of experience as an informational source. We can be aware of the sheer complexity of experience, that "what counts as experience is neither self-evident nor straightforward; it is always contested and always therefore political" (Scott 1991, 797). Whatever it "really" is, it will never be entirely knowable through any of the methodologies or theories available to us, but it remains analytically useful to break it down into *categories* of process that are to a greater or lesser extent conscious or unconscious, predominantly biological or predominantly social, or more to do with perception or with interpretation. Later chapters adopt Bourdieusian, phenomenological, cognitive science, and narrative frameworks because I find each of them helpful in the way they highlight distinct dimensions of experience, but it will always be kept in mind that they are being considered as discrete here for analytic purposes only. The reality of experience, even of the bits that we label "moral," is much less tidy.

From the perspective of the strong version of the social model of disability, which I consider in more detail in chapter 2, a phenomenological approach has a further flaw. Social models of disability redirect the analytic gaze away from the pathologized individual and toward social practices. Paying close attention to the lived experience of being (in) a different kind of body runs counter to this. It puts the "problem" of disability back in the individual and in doing so, critics say, it simply distracts from the real issue, which is that societies incapacitate people who are different. Phenomenological work also pays attention to details of difference, and for many in the disability movement this is problematic in another way. Chapter 2 discusses in more detail recent critiques that argue the strong social model tries to strengthen its case artificially by avoiding the salience of differences between impairments, even though "it is clear that different impairments . . . have different implications for health and individual capacity, [and] also generate different responses from the broader cultural and social milieu" (Shakespeare and Watson 2001). Strong social modellists think that a focus on impairment deflects attention from the systematic ways in which the material and social environment disables people. In reply, social-relationists counter that attending to disability solely as a form of social oppression risks forgetting that "we all live our lives in bodies of a certain sort, whose possibilities and vulnerabilities" belong to the body as much as they belong to the society in which those bodies exist (Nussbaum 1995, 76). (It also, as we shall see, ignores the possibility that not all disabled people are materially oppressed in the way the strong social model thinks.)

Still another theoretical issue is knowing how far knowledge of one individual's lifeworld can be extrapolated to the lives of others. Exploring one person's experience might tell us a lot about a sample group of one, but what does it say about anyone else? At one extreme, the knowledge held by the individual bearer of a unique combination of events and circumstances becomes so unique that it cannot be parlayed into any generalized social statement: idiographic insight reaches "a point where the connection between those experiences and the outside world is not easy to see" (Williams 2001, 137). The best phenomenological and existential phenomenological work, though, does not lose sight of the world beyond the subject. Like any experience, the personal experience of disability is embedded in a common moral world. Paradoxically then, the immersion in local moral worlds, attending closely to what is at stake in the experience of others, is also a way into the shared elements of moral experience.

By concentrating on the empirical and phenomenal understanding of disabled bodies I am trying to put right what I see as a neglect of an important source of insight into real moral lives. It's not a claim that empirical data are the only true source material for thinking about disability, nor that a deeper knowledge of disabled experience will automatically help to craft a disability ethics to which every right-thinking person would agree. The bodies of everyday disabled experience form only part of the knowledge that, along with bodies present in medical discourse, and their representations in popular culture, contributes to the contemporary meaning of abnormality and disability. How being physically unusual affects a person's moral understandings will depend on how it affects her life, and that in turn will depend on the cultural meanings and values that it carries. It will also reflect the ways these meanings and values are modified by biological, material, and symbolic interactions between the individual and society, *and* how each individual makes sense of these interactions for herself, *and* what happens as these microlevel hermeneutics, eventually, feed back into collective understandings.

I will be arguing that to comprehend the disabled body more fully requires following the body through its common and statistically more unusual limitations. One point I want to flag early is that doing so will very probably lead us away from a consistently negative attitude to anomalous embodiment. While only a slavish commitment to ideology would permit anyone to claim that bodily anomaly is *never* a source of difficulty and frustration, it is also true that the experience of embodied difference is not always straightforwardly bad. Corporeally anomalous people are of course different, because that's what being anomalous means, but difference need not always be a *problem*. By definition my own hearing impairment affects my relationship to sound. It also affects how I deal with space, light, noisy neighbors, air travel, being underwater, playing the saxophone, and men whose faces are obscured by their beards. Being deaf has, at times, influenced my evaluation of family and community ties, the obligations of the state to its citizens, and the value of organic matter compared to artificial aids to hearing. I usually find these effects more interesting and complicated than the simple not-being-able-to-hear that the hearing world takes as the essential fact of deafness. None of them are just side effects of my hearing impairment. They are constitutive of my experience of deafness, and as constitutive of my identity as is being a woman or being of mixed race.

Bioethicists should really be interested in disability not because it is a problem to be solved by medical or other means (although sometimes it is that), but because of its capacity to make all of us think differently, and harder. Gelya Frank writes that "truly physically variant human beings challenge the conventional boundaries between male and female, sexed and sexless, animal and human, large and small, and self and other" (Frank 1986, 215–16). Physically unusual people demand justification of deeply held beliefs about how people should be. Thinking seriously and ethically about disability therefore means looking critically at things like bodies and experience that are normally taken for granted, and that some people have a vested interest in taking for granted.

A final few words on what this book does and does not try to do. Most of the discussion concerns physical impairment. The effects of intellectual and cognitive impairment or mental illness on perception and reasoning appear more obvious, and have certainly been more extensively discussed. Because I am chiefly concerned with how embodied, physical anomaly can affect moral perception and reasoning, I do not give much attention to nonphysical impairment or illness. Some of what I have to say, for example about social interactions, is relevant to these kinds of impairment too. However, when it comes to effects on moral judgment I think that learning disabilities and mental illness pose some distinctive questions of their own, and I have neither space nor competence to do proper justice to them here. The risk is of implying a starker mind/body dichotomy than I would wish to.

I also say rather little about carers until chapter 8's discussion of dependencies. In part this is because the role of care in disability and elsewhere has been addressed more extensively by feminist bioethicists (Kittay 1999; Silvers 1995). It will become clear, I hope, that a proper understanding of disability depends on taking into account the full range of perspectives on it, and therefore not excluding (as some disability theorists do) or forgetting (as some bioethicists do) people who are only indirectly touched by impairment. But including all perspectives in a book of this kind would be a hugely ambitious undertaking, and I'm not that reckless.

Some readers may be disappointed that I don't provide a firm conclusion on, say, the ethics of PGD for late-onset disorders, or medical interventions to delay the maturation of children with multiple impairments. My response here is that I think bioethics risks producing flawed, superficial, and—at worst—self-serving solutions if it fails *first of all* to engage more closely with experienced impairment. For that reason, and for the sake of giving a broad view, I've also tried to resist the temptation to follow in detail any one pressing bioethical issue, with the exception of the particular example of chapter 4. Above all, what I hope to do is raise some of the questions I find interesting in disability, and point to directions I would like to see both disability theory and bioethics exploring—preferably in collaboration.

NOTES

1. Biomedicine has also, notoriously, taken an active part in programs of euthanasia of disabled people in the mid-twentieth century. I'm talking here about medical interventions that are broadly accepted as ethically and socially legitimate.

2. As is becoming apparent in the ethical conundrums raised by contemporary cyber and virtual forms of social interaction.

3. There is as yet not much literature on this. A personal account of "normal" pregnancy by a disabled activist can be found in Finger (1990) and also in Lapper (2005).

2

Conceptualizing Disability

It is the theory that decides what can and cannot be observed.

—Einstein to Heisenberg

Simo Vehmas puts it succinctly, if a little bluntly: "The relationship between bioethics and disability has traditionally focused on killing" (Vehmas 2003, 146). By any standards this is a narrow focus. Bioethicists have mostly been called upon (or felt obliged) to evaluate ethically and help regulate the new medical technologies of prenatal or preimplantation screening for impairments, and the voluntary or involuntary euthanasia of disabled people. Combined with its symbiotic relationship with biomedicine, this limited range of tasks has meant that bioethics reflexively turns to the conceptual frameworks of medicine for thinking about disability. In a medical framework, what I will call the *bad thing* of disability—whatever it is that makes being disabled undesirable—is connected in a linear fashion to a clinically identifiable abnormality. This is not necessarily wrong, but it does represent only one idea about disability. With few exceptions, there has been little systematic reflection on whether this theory is the most suitable to answer bioethics' questions about disability—whether, in fact, sticking resolutely to it prevents bioethics from asking different or more interesting ones.

Adopting a medicalized way of thinking means that bioethicists generally do not unpack what they mean by disability. At best they give an undernourished account of it. For example, Peter Singer, probably best known for his controversial work on the ethics of treating newborn disabled infants, sometimes refers very specifically to infants with Down syndrome and spina bifida, but in much of his work uses general descriptions such as "severely

19

handicapped infants" (Kuhse and Singer 1985). In a further example, a recent paper directly contesting social conceptions of disability defines disabled people as those who are deprived by their "constitution" of "worthwhile experience" (Harris 2000, 97). As Steven Edwards points out (2005, 30–31), the problem with this is that there are all sorts of worthwhile experiences that, for reasons at least partly constitutional, some people have and others do not, such as being insensitive to the pleasures of atonal music. But although people who really don't get the point of *Erwartung* may be considered unlucky, they cannot reasonably be called disabled without making the concept of disability uselessly broad. Moreover, Harris' definition, and others used implicitly or explicitly by bioethicists, generally give no weight to subjective accounts of disability, so (for example) they cannot help sort out situations in which people who would conventionally be considered disabled claim that they are perfectly fine as they are, or that the *bad thing* about their impairment is not the particular deprivation other people say it is, but something else.

In my experience many bioethicists are unaware of the range of conceptualizations of disability that other disciplines use. Especially where these conceptualizations have been grounded in the subjective experience of disability, they may be better placed to give a nuanced picture of how disability arises and what is undesirable about it than are purely medical ones. While disability studies offers theoretically sophisticated models, however, they are not always easily integrated into the work of bioethics. As a background to the rest of the book, this chapter considers some of these different tools for thinking about disability, taking a look at their strengths and weaknesses.

We all have an idea in our heads of "disability," the details of which depend on factors like the contact (or lack of it) we have had with disabled people, books we've read, films we've seen, or the presence of disabled people in the community in which we live. For many British people at the start of the twenty-first century, for instance, the idea of blindness was strongly associated with David Blunkett, a prominent Labour politician with a visual impairment who held the office of Home Secretary between 2001 and 2004.[1]

Despite its apparent obviousness, thinking about disability is actually profoundly difficult, because:

1. Any concept of disability has to cope with the enormous *heterogeneity* of impairment.
2. There is disagreement about *what is actually disabling*: is it the biological anomaly, or social responses to it, or something about the interaction of the two, and if so, what?

3. The *language* available for discussing disability is impoverished and forces us to think about it in limited ways.
4. We have relatively little empirical or phenomenological knowledge of the *experience* of disability.

As the paucity of systematic knowledge about the subjective experience of disability is one of the central themes of this book, I will not be considering the last point in any depth here. The rest of this chapter looks at the problems presented by disability's heterogeneity, theorization, and language.

HETEROGENEITY

Any concept of disability should pick out what is distinctive about it (whatever it is that enables us to put one person into the category while another stays outside). But disability is an organizing idea that has to hold together a daunting variety of body states, some universally agreed to be disabling, and others whose status is more contested: sensory impairments, mobility restrictions, missing or lost limbs, skeletal dysplasias (including restricted growth), morphological anomalies ranging from conjoined twins to extra toes, genetic syndromes with complex phenotypes, cognitive impairments and learning difficulties, mental illnesses, disablement due to chronic illness such as HIV/AIDS or metabolic dysfunction, and neurofunctional disorders. The concept of disability also has to cover impairments with different origins: an arm can be missing because someone was born without it, lost it in an accident, or had it amputated to prevent the spread of cancer. It must also include impairments, like spinal cord lesion, that are present all the time; those that are intermittent, such as multiple sclerosis; and others that get progressively worse, like osteoarthritis. And it has to account for the fact that there are people with the *same* bodily variation who disagree on whether they are disabled at all.

All this heterogeneity makes problematic the philosophical habit of invoking an abstract "disability" without saying exactly what kinds of body are involved. Indisputably, the lives of a paraplegic wheelchair user, a signing Deaf person, an adult with Down syndrome, or an infant with the metabolic disorder Gaucher syndrome are significantly different due to the *specific* nature of their impairment. At least some of these differences will be relevant to the judgments that bioethics wants to make about their quality of life—whether other embodiments would be preferable, whether termination of a fetus with the condition is ethically justifiable, and so on.

Some people might object that if in practice we intuitively know what disability is, there is no need to define it. This Wittgensteinian approach (I can't tell you what the word means but I know it when I see it) has the appeal of pragmatism, and in everyday, small-scale encounters we may not need anything more. Still, there are important areas of contemporary life that demand clear definitions of disability. A government agency needs to have a knowledge of disability demographics if it wants to provide adequate social support or services, or to identify where disabled people are being excluded from economic and social participation. Getting this knowledge requires being able to count how many disabled people there are, which means knowing what we are supposed to be counting. A workable definition of disability is needed so that services or benefits in limited supply can be directed to the right people. In Britain, for example, many parents of children with impairment fight to have them given a "statement of special educational needs," known colloquially as "being statemented," because this is the key to getting educational support for their child. And definitions are of course crucial in the familiar bioethical terrain of prenatal or preimplantation diagnosis of disability and in end-of-life decisions, although the legal wording is often kept deliberately vague here to leave room for case-by-case interpretation.

THEORIES AND MODELS

Disability as Individual Trouble: Moral and Medical

The category of "the disabled" seems to be a recent one (Braddock and Parish 2001; Borsay 2005). Before the nineteenth century, impairments such as blindness, deafness, lameness, or madness appeared as distinct states and were not gathered under a single label. It has been suggested that the grouping together was primarily a bureaucratic convenience, driven by a post-Enlightenment desire to make society orderly at a time when the increasing ability of life science to describe human bodily standards resulted in more and more nonstandard forms being cataloged (Feinstein 1975; Helman 1990), and when social policy in Britain and the United States was beginning to provide for the poor who "deserved" support because their inability to work was a result of impairment (Barnes, et al. 1999, 18–20; Oliver 1990). In parallel with administrative moves to gather impairments under a single heading, ideas about the constitution and cause of impairment have generally focused on things going wrong with the individual. In prescientific societies, disability is frequently taken as a punishment for moral or religious transgression. Although transgression may be collective as well as individual, in that a person may suffer as a consequence of *community* or ancestral wrongdoing (as in the doctrine of original sin), moral models like these more often involve individuals who have done wrong and who receive their just deserts in the form of a dodgy leg.

In contemporary life, biomedicine has taken over from religion ... ing to offer the best response to illness and disability. Although this is usually referred to as "the medical model," that term can be misleading: it is not necessarily the view that any doctor will hold, and in any case there is more than one way of modeling disability in medical terms, in line with the methodological diversity of medicine itself. Broadly, the key feature of a medicalized view is that disability is a nominative pathology: a defect or deficit located in an individual. What counts as defect or deficit is determined by reference to a norm of physical or mental structure and function. The parameters of the norm are given by biomedical science, which since the eighteenth century has increasingly been concerned with quantifying deviation. So from a medicalized perspective, disability is an abnormality of form or function, the cause of which lies in the biology of the individual. For their part, bioethicists have been inclined to accept biomedicine's delineations of the norms of human embodiment. Although biomedicine often gives a role to nonmedical factors in contributing to *causing* disability, it generally does not implicate the environment or social-world in the *constitution* of disability, as social-relational models do.

This brief description necessarily caricatures medicine's take on disability to some degree. But allowing for some overgeneralization, I think it still reflects quite accurately the dominant ethos in medicine—and therefore in mainstream bioethics too.

Disability as Individual Trouble: Genetic

Recent advances in genetic medicine and the efforts of the Human Genome Project (HGP) (Watson and Cook-Deegan 1991; Judson 1992; Kevles 1992) have resulted in a genetic version of the medical model of disability. I want to spend a little time on this, not because genetic explanations for impairment are necessarily the best or the most relevant, but because the current explanatory power of genetics means that its accounts of disability are disproportionately influential and so warrant special attention.

Genetic ideas are variously implicated in disability. The inheritance patterns of familial disorders have been traced and used for decades to provide counseling for reproductive decisions. Genetic testing allows individuals carrying specific genes to be identified, prenatally or postnatally, their symptoms matched to genetic diagnoses, and in an increasing number of cases gene loci have been identified to the extent that prenatal genetic testing and preimplantation genetic diagnosis are possible. Some of the pathology-related genes identified are associated with predispositions to the later development of disabling conditions, raising some difficult ethical and practical questions about whether the possession of a characteristic genotype (the genetic makeup) in the absence of an effect on phenotype[2] (morphology or function) counts as an impairment.

The image of the relationship between genes and phenotype that currently dominates our thinking is linear and deterministic. In this "program" model of gene action, the DNA sequences of an organism are responsible for phenotypic characteristics and therefore for all human variation. Thus the foundational cause of disability is found encoded in the gene sequences that give rise, in a predictable manner, to a particular disabling bodily variation. This reductionist and determinist paradigm of gene action has gained support from the sequencing of the human genome, which is (wrongly) taken to mean that there is "a" normal human genome rather than numerous normalities. Phenotypic abnormality is increasingly interpreted as reflecting deviation from the canonical genomic norm and is taken as indicating the possession of a defective genome. The criticisms that have been levelled by social scientists and cultural commentators at this picture of the interaction between gene and organism are well known, and I will not repeat them here. In fact molecular biologists now consider this to be an inaccurate portrayal of gene function (Oyama et al. 2003; Neumann-Held and Rehmann-Sutter 2006). This is why I have argued elsewhere (Scully 2002, 2006a) that molecular biology actually provides material for a deeper questioning of the norms of embodiment. Although medical practice is structured by a normal/pathological dichotomy, genetic models of human variation can be used without necessarily supporting such binary oppositions between normal and abnormal. Within molecular and developmental biology there exist a number of alternative, non-program models that relate gene expression to developmental processes and the maintenance of organism systems (Griffiths and Neumann-Held 1999). Such processual or systems approaches break down the dichotomy between genetic information and the organism's phenotype, and embodiment becomes "an autonomous developmental process which is not separate from psychic and mental and social development" (Rehmann-Sutter 2002, 46).

In the previous chapter I contrasted the two frameworks that dominate theorizing about the body, the postmodern and the genetic. While postmodern frameworks destabilize a normative ideal by fundamentally rejecting both the metanarrative of normalization and the whole idea of a stable and coherent subject, genetic frameworks—paradoxically—can be used to do something similar. In the early twentieth century, the science of genetics was more interested in the association of different kinds of phenotype with genotype, and less in the detection of deviation from the normal. That means that geneticists needed genetic and phenotypic diversity (the more the merrier) to build genetic theory, and because of that were receptive to the view that genotypic "normality" always encompasses a wide spread of states. Although on the surface this is a small difference, it is crucial because it effectively resists classifying variations as normal/abnormal. As long as the temptation to compare genetic variation with a genomic norm can be resisted, then the diversity of individual sequence data, which becomes obvious as soon as we start to collect it, offers a way of talking about variation that changes the whole conceptualization of genotypic and phenotypic difference.

Disability as Social Relation: The Strong Social Model

Alternatives to the individual, usually medical, framework come under the broad heading of social models of disability (Abberley 1987; Oliver 1990, 1996; Barnes 1998; Linton 1998; Shakespeare 2006). One version has been so prominent (and caused so much contention) that it is often referred to as "the" social model. I refer to it here as the "strong social model," since I find it more helpful to take a range of ways of thinking about disability as social or social-relational. Social-relational models suggest that disability is a product of the interaction, at personal and structural levels, between physical or mental anomaly and the social world in which someone lives (Thomas 2007, 52). Where the models differ is in exactly how they describe the interaction between the two and the kind of problems they see being generated as a result. → created b/c didn't account for privilege gaps

The strong social model originated within British disability activism in the 1970s and 1980s, when disability activist groups became dissatisfied with the inability of a purely medical perspective to take into account the social and economic features that, they felt, conspired to produce disability (Oliver 1990; Campbell and Oliver 1996; Shakespeare 2006; Thomas 2007). The strong social model is a structural analysis of disability as a phenomenon generated by social organizations that discriminate against some embodiments. Its fundamental critique is that medicalized thinking confuses the *bad thing* of disability with the phenotypic crossing of a biological limit. In the redefinition of disability published in 1976 by one group of activists, the Union of the Physically Impaired Against Segregation (UPIAS), disability was effectively separated from the body, breaking the conflation of impairment and disability on which the medical framework relies. While *impairment* in the strong social model is an individual biological manifestation such as hearing loss, *disability* is the "disadvantage . . . caused by a contemporary social organization which takes no or little account of people who have physical impairments and hence excludes them from participation in the mainstream of social activities. Physical disability is therefore a particular form of social oppression" (UPIAS 1976, 14). Accordingly, it is barriers to participation in society, and especially to participation in the labor market, which are disabling—not any intrinsic property of the body. From this perspective the strong social model advocates removing socioeconomic barriers to civil participation before anything else.[3]

The strong social model has been a major influence in disability theory, in shaping disability activism's political demands, and in helping many disabled people rethink the meaning of disability in their lives, as I describe in chapter 7. It nevertheless faces strong criticism from both within and beyond disability studies. In focusing exclusively on the material basis of disability, some strong social modelists appear to suggest that the *bad thing* of disability has little or nothing at all to do with bodily variation. The disadvantage that constitutes disability could be eradicated if the appropriate modifications were made to modes of production, architecture, transport, information provision, and education. Then although impairments would remain, they would not be impediments in people's lives because the barriers that create disablement would have gone.

While this could be true for some, perhaps even many, impairments, it does not plausibly account for all of them or all their multiple effects. My life would be a lot more like other people's if aids to hearing, like induction loops, were routinely installed (and properly maintained) in all buildings and if all public announcements were made visually as well as aurally. This would be a removal of environmental barriers that block my full participation in activities that other, hearing people engage in. But I don't see that any amount of environmental rearrangement will do much to alleviate the intermittent tinnitus I get, which is an indisputably negative effect (only someone who really likes the sound of dried peas pouring onto a metal roof could not consider it negative) and one that is intrinsic to my hearing impairment.

Medical theory has made some attempt to accommodate the insights of social-relational models of disability, including the terminology of impairment, but without fully adopting the distinctive materialist construction of disability that the strong social model advocates. For example, the World Health Organization has produced two typologies of disability, twenty years apart, and with subtle differences in key categories. The 1980 International Classification of Impairments, Disabilities and Handicaps (ICIDH) distinguishes among impairment, disability, and handicap (WHO 1980). Impairment is defined as "any loss or abnormality of psychological, physiological or anatomical structure or function"; impairments give rise to disabilities, which are "any restriction or lack . . . of ability to perform an activity in the manner or within the range considered normal for a human being"; and both impairments and disabilities can lead to handicap, "a disadvantage . . . that limits or prevents the fulfilment of a role that is normal (depending on age, sex and cultural factors) for that individual." So instead of presenting a purely medical picture, the ICIDH recognizes disadvantage resulting from the interaction of the impaired biological substrate and the social world. However, it is quite a different kind of interaction from that invoked by versions of the social-relational model that see the interface between impairment and surroundings actively generating disability, whether through marginalizing social barriers or discriminatory cultural representations. The ICIDH invokes social factors in the context of the individual's failure to fit an expected social role.

Twenty years later, and partly as a response to criticism from disability scholars and activists, the WHO's revised classificatory system, the International Classification of Functioning, Disability and Health (ICF), replaced the previous categories with the new ones of impairment, activity limitations, and participation restrictions (WHO 2001). Although the headings have changed, the formal structure is still the same. But unlike the ICIDH, the ICF states explicitly that disability is "a dynamic interaction" (WHO 2001, 10) between diseases and disorders (factors intrinsic to the individual) and contextual factors, the nature of which are determined by the culture or society in which the individual lives. So although the ICF clearly does not adopt the strong social model of disability, the influence of social-relational thinking is apparent. The authors of the ICF felt it necessary to acknowledge nonbiological factors contributing to the experience of disability. Still, the ICF remains a typology, not a theory of disability: it has a "background theory" which recognizes that organ impairment, organismic function, and social organization all play a part in disability, but it goes no further than that.

The strong social model has been taken to task by myself and other disability scholars, many of whom write from an explicitly feminist perspective, for its neglect of the nonmaterial aspects of disability. The strong social model is just not that interested in the subjective experience of the impaired body, or its psychoemotional aspects, or the processes through which disability is constructed by cultural representations and language.[4] Its separation of impairment and disability, useful in refocusing attention on the material part of the interaction between the individual and the outside world, means that strong social modelists find paying attention to impairment itself counterproductive. They have argued that theorizing impairment in any way is harmful because it reintroduces the idea that impairment per se is important to the experience of disability. Some theorists suggest that the strong social model's reluctance to take seriously the embodied reality of impairment stems from the fear that admitting a level of irremovable difficulty in impairment might compromise the nondisabled world's will, not great at the best of times, to make the necessary social modifications to remove disabling barriers. The strong social model's recalcitrance has some basis in academic territorialism as well, because as Carol Thomas notes, "Disability studies made its way into the academy on the basis of its opposition to the idea, deeply rooted both within and outside social science disciplines, that 'disability' and 'being disabled' is *all about* the body and its defects" (Thomas 2007, 121).

Its historical materialism makes the strong social model equally unsym-pathetic to the role of discourse in disability or impairment. Poststruc-turalist disability theorists, however, hold that the removal of the kind of structural barriers that strong social modellists worry about would leave in-tact "the attitudinal and discursive dimensions of social relations," which they argue are just as effective as the more tangible ones at marginalizing disabled people and blocking the political goals of the disability move-ment (Hughes 2002). Indeed, poststructuralists find the strong social model as guilty of perpetuating false dichotomies as the biomedical. As we've seen, the actual mode of operation of medicalized thinking is a bi-nary one in which the standard of normative embodiment is imposed against the "chaotic residue" (Griffiths 1995, 171) of all the other embod-iments that fail to match up. Poststructuralism sees something similar go-ing on in the binary split between impairment and disability in the strong social model. And poststructuralists join with phenomenological critics of the strong social model in saying that it not only reinforces the traditional Cartesian dualism of the mind/body split, but its dismissal of the impaired body effectively concedes it to biomedicine. If social-relational approaches have nothing to say about impairment, then biomedicine will have every-thing to say about it.

Aside from the strong social model's strategic flaws, the conceptual accu-racy of its binary split between impairment and disability has also been called into question. There is an analogy here with the separation of sex and gender in feminist theory. For feminist thinking in the 1970s and 1980s, it was analytically invaluable to be able to consider the biological nature of the sexed body separately from the gendering of social roles, that is, taking sex/gender as one manifestation of the nature/culture couple. By the 1990s, however, many feminist philosophers were following Judith Butler (1990, 6–9, 36–38) in arguing that the line between the two was not as clear as it had seemed. The discursive paradigm suggested that not even the biology of the body presents to us "as is"—we can only comprehend biology be-cause of the discursive tools with which culture equips us. Our grasp of "bi-ological sex" is a form of culturally mediated understanding, just as much as more obviously socially constructed gender roles are. In a similar way, poststructuralist disability theorists suggest, it is never possible for us as hu-man observers to get a view of the body and its variations from outside, be-fore or beyond language, because it is only through language that we can make sense of it in the first place. Poststructuralist theorists hold that lan-guage and representation are important routes to understanding the onto-logical and moral meaning of disability in the modern, discourse-saturated world. In the extreme, some poststructuralist writing about disability, tak-ing the disabled self as a discursively constructed social identity, seems to be saying that it is discursive practices *alone* that make a person disabled.

More plausibly perhaps, Corker, throughout her work, discusses disability not as created by discourse, but as having features, ignored by the social model's focus on material barriers, that operate through language. I will return to a consideration of linguistic issues shortly.

Other Social-Relational Approaches

The strong social model does not exhaust the possibilities of social-relational thinking about disability. Others include the minority model, most strongly advocated in North America, which sees disabled people as a minority group in relation to majority society. It is "clear about the role of the social environment" in creating minority status (Shakespeare 2006, 24), and as a consequence it focuses on achieving civil rights legislation to fight prejudice and discrimination. Other social-relational approaches have been methodologically more inclined toward engaging with subjective experience and the representation of the impaired body. Here, feminists in disability studies have been foremost in resisting attempts to separate the domains of private experience and public oppression, arguing that while it is sometimes analytically useful, in the end such splitting leads to a substantial depletion of disability theory. The marginalization of disabled people cannot be effectively tackled, either theoretically or politically, if the subjective experience of impairment is left out. Liz Crow has written that disabled women's need "to find a way to integrate impairment into our whole experience and sense of ourselves" is not solely for the benefit of their own sense of integrity, but on behalf of "our individual and collective capacity to work against disability" (Crow 1996, 210).

To acknowledge the intrinsic disadvantage of some impairments without diluting the strong social model's analytic strengths, Carol Thomas introduced the term *impairment effects* for the restrictions of activity or behavior that can be traced back directly to bodily impairments and therefore might be called "biological." However, Thomas also wants to understand the body as "simultaneously biological, material and social" (2007, 135), and so suggests that even this apparently straightforward biological/social dualism cannot be sustained, because the activities that are restricted and the norm against which the body is compared are both socially contingent. Abnormalities of body form, for instance, are less common in advanced industrial societies than in rural or preindustrial ones, for social reasons to do with better healthcare and accident prevention. A limb abnormality in contemporary society is understood against a historically specific background of norms, frequency and type of abnormalities, beliefs about the etiology and meaning of the impairment, and so on. As Thomas says, "in any 'real' social setting, impairments, impairment effects and disablism are thoroughly intermeshed with the social conditions that bring them into being and give them meaning" (2007, 137). That meaning informs our ethical judgment of impairment and has an ethical component too.

PHENOTYPIC VARIATION

In each of the models of disability just sketched out, the term *impairment* has a distinct place and significance. In the classic medical model, impairment is used interchangeably with phenotypic variation and disability. In the ICIDH, impairment is "any loss or abnormality of psychological, physiological or anatomical structure or function," and it has a causal relationship to disability and handicap. The ICF definition is similar, although the relationship between the "loss or abnormality" of impairment and activity or participation limitations is more tentative. And in the UPIAS definition adopted by the strong social model, impairment is the state of "lacking part or all of a limb, or having a defective limb, organ or mechanism of the body" (UPIAS 1976; Oliver 1990, 11).

Whatever function or place it takes in a theory of disability, the word *impairment* has a specific meaning (in English): *to impair* is *to reduce or weaken in strength, quality, etc.*[5] The definition does not include the possibility of a morphological or functional variation that does *not* have a harmful impact on the "strength, quality, etc." on the limb or organ and/or on the subjective experience of the individual. This is a significant gap because there needs to be space in which to describe a variation in body form or function prior to making judgments about its effects.

Ironically, the genetic model may be the one that can most easily do this (although as discussed earlier, it tends not to be used that way). Geneticists know that many mutations or changes in DNA sequences either have no effect on the structure of the resulting protein (because of the redundancy of the genetic code), or the effect does not detectably alter its function. And even if the genotypic change does alter the protein, the change in phenotype may not significantly affect the organism's *biological* functioning. Biologists are most interested in the biological characteristics on which natural selection operates. But for humans living in complex social groups where the direct effects of natural selection are largely buffered, an even greater degree of body diversity is neutral in its effect on a person's life. At some point, phenotypic diversity becomes problematic for the individual; where and why this happens is not solely the result of the magnitude of the divergence from the norm, but also the nature of the interaction between the phenotype and the surrounding conditions.

It may be helpful then to use "phenotypic variation" to distinguish the deviation from species-typicality, before we start to measure how much of an *impairment* the deviation is. This is similar to Thomas' distinction between impairment and impairment effects, but I think her use of "impairment" here jumps the gun. "Phenotypic variation" takes longer to say, but it allows us to start from all physicalities and *then* see which are actively disadvantageous. Saying that a phenotypic variation is not equivalent to impairment is not to trivialize or ignore the very real difficulties associated with certain physical variations. However, separating phenotypic variation and impairment has the advantage that the distinct criteria by which each is identified and evaluated can also be differentiated. Being able to do this is important—not just analytic hairsplitting—because otherwise the number of *surrogates* that are involved slips out of sight.

What I mean by this is that the *bad thing* of disability is not in practice the loss or malfunction of a body part or system. When making judgments about quality of life, or appropriate interventions—the kind of judgments bioethics makes—we are not that interested in how well an organ or biochemical pathway works. These things are relevant to the ethical judgments only by virtue of their impact on the life in question. A disabled person *suffers*, if she suffers, from particular subjective experiences of pain, disadvantage, difficulty, or exclusion, which are undesirable. The details of these experiences, including how severe the effect is and what aspects of life are affected, will differ from person to person according to individual circumstances and context. Usually, however, we don't examine the details. What we do is take one step back from the lived experience and insert the idea of impairment to "stand for" the experience of pain, disadvantage, and so on: impairment is used as a surrogate marker for the set of experiences we call disability. But surrogate markers are stand-ins, not the thing itself. If we take the argument of social-relational models and say that the connection between impairment and the experience of disablement is dependent on social-environmental factors and therefore is not as linear as is commonly assumed, the validity of the surrogate marker, that is, whether it really can stand for disability in that way, becomes more questionable.

The modern biomedical view of disability goes further, taking an additional step back from impairment. Here, a variation in *phenotype* becomes a surrogate marker for *impairment*. Now as we've discussed, simple phenotypic variation is not always disadvantageous either biologically or socially.[6] As biological and social beings we live immersed in phenotypic variations, some of which stand out. Sometimes they stand out because they really do have major impairment effects (you'd be hard pressed to argue that the absence of limbs is not impairing in some degree). In practice, however, rather than evaluate *how* impairing a phenotypic variation is in each case, it is simpler just to look out for unfamiliar variants. Physical variations that we encounter often will tend to be thought of as lying within the normal range, while those that are statistically more unusual will not be. In the first instance, then, what we actually spot as impairment is not a biological or social "reduction in quality," but the individual's match to the human phe-notypic norm. We recognize that having only one arm rather than two in a world of shoelaces is definitely impairing, but would not think of suggest-ing that having only two arms rather than three is an impairment, even though we also live in a world where small children and shopping have to be carried at the same time as we search a pocket for the front-door keys; having three arms would then be rather useful. The assumption that unfa-miliar kinds of variation are impairing forecloses our examination of whether this is true, and if so whether it is the degree of variation itself or the particular social and cultural responses it elicits that makes it true.

The advent of the genomic body introduces yet another level of surro-gacy. Here, it's an alteration of the DNA sequence that is taken as an ade-quate and reliable predictor of a subsequent change in phenotype. I noted earlier the need to be cautious about making this assumption, given the cur-rent limits to genetic knowledge and the fact that, if the systems theories of gene action are correct, the outcome of DNA sequence changes at the level of the organism may be inherently unpredictable. The identification of a person as disabled *on the basis of* his or her genotype is a radical shift in the meaning of both disability and impairment. It takes chemically encoded in-formation as a suitable marker for phenotypic change, and then for im-paired structure and function, and then for the lived experience of disad-vantage. The process begins to look like a set of Russian dolls, each one step further removed from the *bad thing* of disability that worried us in the first place.

It is important to emphasize here that my argument is not that such sur-rogate markers can never be used. Genetic mutations do often lead to phe-notypic variation; phenotypic variation is often impairing; impairments fre-quently lead to experienced disablement. But the use of surrogates always carries the risk of confusing the marker with the thing itself, and of not noticing the instances where the surrogacy is invalid. It is legitimate to use the surrogate markers of disability discourse in the way I described as long as we are conscious of what we are doing, and as long as scrupulous atten-tion is paid to the limits of each marker's ability to represent its target. This degree of scrupulousness (or pedantry) is uncommon in bioethical writing on disability.

LANGUAGE

Unfortunately, the difficulty of agreeing on what constitutes disability is compounded by the language we use. Some of the clarifications of vocabu-lary I have outlined above are extremely useful: defining terms precisely and using them with care are conducive to clarity of thought, and in general it

is helpful to be able to think our way as clearly as possible through a phenomenon as complex as disability. The rigor with which the strong social
model reserves "impairment" for the biological anomaly and "disability"
for the experience of oppression and social exclusion can seem irritatingly
picky, but is invaluable in parsing the types of effects belonging to each domain, and for spotting where it really is impossible to disentangle them
completely. It is less helpful when analytical rigor turns into a party line
about details of vernacular; most disability scholars I know would be happy
never to sit through another argument about whether it is proper to refer to
"disabled people," as the British disability movement does, or "people with
disabilities," commoner in the U.S. people-first movement. (For the record,
throughout this book I generally use "disabled people" because it is the
form I am most used to, and I use "disability" fairly loosely to refer to all
aspects of it, except where I use "impairment" specifically to highlight the
phenotypic element over the social.)

A more intractable problem, however, is the overall lack of neutral language to discuss disability. This is a difficulty that extends from the most
crass pejorative slang about disabled people, down to the discursive structure
of social categories. Problems of the first kind are much easier to spot. The
words people elect to use demonstrate their respect, or lack of it, for members of other groups. This matters because particular words cause offense, to
women or ethnic minorities, for example, but also because their use engen-
ders alienation, contempt, or hatred in those who use them. We may not
want to go so far as to say that language constructs our attitudes, but it seems
plausible that whenever we opt unchallenged for one term over another, the
cognate attitudes are reinforced. Awareness of this process is an additional
reason why sexist and racist words have become gradually unacceptable, and
so have terms like "cripple," "deaf and dumb," and "mongol." Nevertheless,
changes in vocabulary will solve the problem only if contempt, hate, fear,
and so on are *solely* generated through people's choice of words, rather than
the words' also being a reflection of underlying attitudes. This is what lies behind the well-recognized effect of "creeping stigmatization," where persistent and unacknowledged prejudices manage to contaminate novel, supposedly value-neutral terminology. An especially florid example here is the
lengthy list of names adopted and discarded for what we currently call "developmental disorders" or "learning difficulties"; terms such as "cretin,"
"moron," "idiot," "mongol," "mentally retarded," "intellectually disabled,"
and "special" have successively become too loaded to use.

One need not be a card-carrying poststructuralist to acknowledge that examining the language of disability is *ethically* important. Language not only
affects the everyday treatment of disabled people, it also determines the
technical capacity to conceptualize in moral terms the agents and situations
that bioethicists discuss. If "wheelchair user" says something significantly

different about the agency of a person than "wheelchair bound" does, for instance; and if constant repetition of "wheelchair bound" or "suffering from/afflicted by multiple sclerosis" subtly reinforces distorting cultural stereotypes of people with that impairment; and if we know all this, then we are morally responsible for the terms we choose to use. The counterside is the importance of not becoming a zealot about wording at the price of forgetting the reasons for it: to improve our ethical analysis, and to resist offensive and damaging stereotyping of disabled people.[7]

Aside from the need to avoid harmful words, and to find the right words to support ethical analysis, disability faces a special structural challenge when it enters into language. Disability is often treated as a category of identifying characteristic, one among other dimensions of social identity along with gender, ethnicity, age, and sexuality. As embodied subjects, people identify themselves and others in terms of these categories. Although each category gathers together all manifestations (that a society recognizes) of the relevant characteristic—so that gender includes a minimum of two manifestations, ethnicity many more—within categories manifestations are also implicitly ranked according to their social status. Within the category of gender, for instance, men and women are differentiated *and* men are generally accorded a higher ranking in line with their social position. These hierarchies are not often made explicit, but they do not need to be: they involve the kind of tacit knowledge about social arrangements that everyone just has.

Disability occupies an anomalous position within the typology of gender, class, ethnicity, sexuality, or age, because unlike any of these it is possible for a person to exist outside the category. One can be not disabled, in a way that one cannot be not gendered, for example, or not have an age or class. As a level of classification, disability seems to be less equivalent to "gender" than it is to, say, "women." Just as it is possible for some gendered people not to be women, it is possible not to be disabled. Disability is a manifestation or subcategory of something more encompassing, as women are a subcategory of the wider concept of gender.[8]

But if that's the case, we have to contend with a real linguistic inadequacy. What word is available that stands in the same relation to being disabled that "gender" signifies in relation to being a woman? English and other European languages, as far as I know, lack a concise way of saying "the general category of characteristics, one manifestation of which is what we mean when we talk about impairment." "Ability" is not adequate here, partly because it is too broad, and partly because it is the negative of disability: it is the equivalent of "not-woman," or man, not of "gender." We might consider "species-typical functioning" (Boorse 1977; Daniels 1987) although that term begs a lot of questions about the limits of species typicality and the meaning of function (Amundsen 2005). "Phenotype" might work, although it is unfamiliar, and it also includes sex/gender or racial characteristics.

There might be better vocabulary, but the point is that we don't go looking for alternatives—disability is the concept we hang on to. In practice that
means that when someone is assigned to the category "disabled," we have
already made a judgment about which of the two possibilities, disabled/not
disabled, she is. For race, let's say, the equivalent is when we note that someone is black and not white. But a conversation about black people (rather
than white people), or about men (rather than women) is a different sort
of conversation from one about gender or one about race. It takes place
within a frame of agreements about relevant facts and possibilities, knowledge of what has already been determined and what is still up for discussion; it foregrounds certain elements and closes off others.

Language forces us to make a preemptive judgment about disability just
in order to talk about it. In the previous chapter I made the point that "disability" and equivalent words (disorder, malfunction, invalid, deformed,
disfigured) are inescapably about negation and wrongness, so that from the
outset the discussion is about a disvalued manifestation of the body, in a
way that the discussion of gender and race are not. While these categories
make judgments of value through the internal ranking of their members,
for disability the category *alone* is an evaluation.

The connotations of inadequacy, deficit, and dependency associated with
disability, which are so stigmatized in contemporary Western culture (Kittay 1999), form a subliminal background to how we think about disabled
people's lives. I think it likely these connotations also color our imagining
of the social roles that disabled people occupy, of their moral competence
and agency, and of the moral relationships that exist between members of
that category and those outside it. At least in academic talk it would be rare
today to challenge openly the moral status of disabled adults, but there are
enough empirical examples of disabled people's wishes being overridden or
their expressed preferences dismissed to indicate that as a group, disabled
people are often held to be less competent moral agents than nondisabled
ones.[9] This does not mean that categorization as "disabled" is *only* ever a
preemptive moral evaluation, or that everyone makes the same kind of
moral evaluation. But if the description of disability takes the form, even
sometimes, of a moral evaluation, then *from the outset* our discussions are
morally as well as biologically, socially, and discursively marked, and this
needs to be taken into account in a bioethical engagement with disability.

BIOETHICS AND DISABILITY THEORY

The contemporary theorists I find most helpful articulate a sense that disability has biological, socioeconomic, discursive, political, cultural, psychological, and moral dimensions, with any one model or theory prioritizing
selected aspects of the whole. Biomedically based models, including genetic

ones, are best able to catalog developmental difference and provide biological mechanisms for it. Social models are best placed to trace the interactions between individual and society, especially the consequences of collective practices. Discursive approaches illuminate the linguistic construction of disability and other dimensions of difference. We can exploit each theoretical approach for what it does best while remaining aware that its perspective is partial, and that there is no reason why all perspectives should fit readily within a single theory of disability.

Bioethics is still most at home with biomedical and life science approaches to disability. This is to be expected: Anglo-American bioethics has principally been interested in the practical questions that disability poses to life sciences rather than its moral or ontological meaning, while the Continental tradition of bioethics, although more inclined to address metaphysical issues of being and finitude, still uses the medical narratives of the body as its starting point. The question then is whether nonbiomedical models of disability offer useful alternatives with which to do bioethical work.

Of all the perspectives considered here, it is hardest to see bioethics working with the strong social model. The problem is that this perspective shifts disability into areas where bioethics has little expertise or experience, and hitherto not much interest either. If the *bad thing* about disability is purely the consequence of social arrangements, then bioethics would have to agree that the ethically appropriate responses to disability lie primarily in the social, economic, or political orders. The ethical debate about the "problem" of disability should not be about regulating reproductive technologies in order to be clear on which fetuses can legitimately be terminated, for example, but about redistributing economic resources, and changing educational and employment policies, to ensure that people with impairment get a fair shot at the goods the rest of society enjoys. This is clearly an ethical and political issue, but not an obviously *bioethical* one. If the strong social model of disability is adopted, there is not much that bioethics can contribute.

However, I think bioethicists are also likely to reject the strong social model for reasons other than a fear of professional futility. They think its materialist focus simply wrong, crude, or misdirected, and as we have seen they would be joined here by disability scholars and activists who find the strong social model incapable of capturing important aspects of disability—as incapable as a purely medical approach, although for different reasons.

Other more culturally oriented methodologies, including feminist, poststructuralist, and broadly postmodern perspectives, already form part (albeit often a marginal one) of the bioethical repertoire. Thus feminist bioethicists have analyzed the representation of gender and authority in reproductive medicine and elsewhere; Foucauldian strategies have been used to trace the routes of "biopower" in contemporary society's use of biomedicine and genetics (Ashcroft 2003, 2005; Frank and Jones 2003; Rabinow and Rose 2006);

and poststructural analyses have been brought to bear on the discursive practices through which biological entities are created (Shildrick 1997; Shildrick and Mykitiuk 2005). All of these offer bioethics useful theoretical traction on disability, such as its representation in biomedical knowledge, the discursive practices that delineate normality/abnormality, or an examination of the disciplinary and self-disciplinary regimes around the social maintenance of certain kinds of body (Tremain 2005). Feminist approaches to bioethics offer perhaps the most accessible bridge between mainstream bioethics and disability studies, by foregrounding the subtle ethical and epistemological effects of social categorization, and through feminism's practice of rigorously scrutinizing power relations. And following feminist ethics, disability ethics knows it must both resist the temptation to oversimplify the real complexity of social identities and find ways to integrate diverse and dynamic notions of disability into ethical analysis.

Theoretical frameworks are developed not to keep theorists occupied, but to help make sense of otherwise chaotic observation and experience. Alongside greater theoretical diversity in its reflections on disability, then, bioethics also needs a more empirically and experientially informed grasp of it. In the next chapter I explore in more detail why that is, and why traditional routes of accommodating the experiences of others are limited.

NOTES

1. Whether this association was particularly helpful to the status of visually impaired people is more questionable, as neither Blunkett nor his policies were universally popular. His guide dogs, however, were held in considerable affection by the British public, with extensive press coverage whenever one of them retired from active service.

2. I introduced the term phenotype in the previous chapter. Although the term is unfamiliar to nonbiologists, I use it throughout this book as a useful, broad, and neutral term to cover the "outcome" organism, the physical and mental characteristics that are the culmination of genetic, cellular, systemic, and environmental contributions.

3. Strictly speaking, by this definition people who are socially marginalized for reasons other than bodily anomaly are also disabled. According to the strong social model, a woman cut off from mainstream social activities because she is unemployed, a single parent, and living on an isolated housing estate may be considered as socially disabled as a wheelchair user.

4. Disability scholarship in the United States has been readier to take a literary or humanities approach here.

5. This definition is taken from the *Collins Concise Dictionary* (1988).

6. I'm referring here to social and cultural forms of disadvantage, but a similar point can be made about biological ones too. In terms of natural selection it is normal, and in fact preferable, for a population to show phenotypic variation. Any real population that does not contain a stock of variety is potentially in deep trouble, as

it has no adaptive flexibility to draw on if its habitat changes. Biologically, there are always phenotypic variations, which at some point become individually maladaptive as those organisms will not survive to reproduce as much as others.

7. In real life, speech and text are not decontextualized, and in context, using the "wrong" language may not indicate a bias against disabled people. Much depends on a speaker's biography, cultural background, and relationship with the listener and with disability (some of the least politically correct language about disability comes from disabled people). Without knowing the context it is hard to be certain whether the language reflects unjust attitudes and, especially, whether it translates into unjust acts. As a disabled colleague once told me unequivocally: "I don't care what they call me as long as they treat me right."

8. One reason why disability is put alongside the others is as a reflection of a minority civil rights model of disability: disability needs to be there because, just as people may be unjustly discriminated against because of their gender, class, race, and so on, they can be discriminated against on the basis of an impairment.

9. This is of course complicated by the fact that for some impairments, notably severe learning difficulties and some forms of mental illness, moral competence genuinely is compromised.

3

Exploring Moral Understandings[1]

> A dialogue which claims absolute understanding of the other is, in effect,
> a monologue which subsumes differences under norms already in place.
> The social fabric may alter as an effect of dialogue and action but the in-
> equalities within it will remain in place.
>
> —Rosalind Diprose

Bioethics is a discipline whose boundaries are not yet firmly set, with an interdisciplinary feel to it (Rothman 1991; Jonsen 1998; Rehmann-Sutter et
al. 2006). It has been described as having been born in the dialogue between practitioners of many disciplines (Borry et al. 2005). Beneath the interdisciplinarity, though, it is recognizably a child of moral philosophy
within the Anglo-American analytic tradition. Most bioethicists probably
feel themselves engaged in a form of philosophical inquiry and not, say, a
sociological one. As it has developed, bioethics has drawn on the numerous
theoretical frameworks developed by moral philosophy for the systematic
analysis of ethical problems. They include the "traditional" theoretical
frameworks of various forms of deontological ethics, utilitarianism and
other consequentialist approaches, ancient and contemporary schools of
virtue ethics, casuistic ethics and their descendants, and contractarian theories. Meanwhile, a bioethical literature is starting to emerge from the non-
traditional approaches of feminist, ethnic, postcolonial, and gay and lesbian ethics.

As branches of applied ethics, medical and bioethics have primarily been
occupied with applying different ethical theories to the practical problems
they confront. Bioethicists have not been overly concerned with metaethi-
cal questions, or with deciding which normative theory is best in general

(although they often have an opinion about that), but rather with which one is most useful for doing the sort of thing bioethics needs to do. I argued in the previous two chapters that bioethics has taken too restricted a view of what it needs to do with and for disability, a myopia reflected in the limited repertoire of analytic procedures and arguments that it has brought to bear on impairment issues, and in a lack of engagement with the conceptual basis of disability.

When I first made the professional transition to bioethics, there was much about philosophy that took me by surprise. High on the list was the absence of an empirical basis for the arguments that moral philosophers made; even stranger was the lack of any apparent felt need for such information. Moral philosophers seem rather ready to offer their reflections as universally representative, and rather unwilling to concede that their points of view might depend on their being the kind of people they (we) are, living the lives they (we) do. This was unnerving for someone trained not to extrapolate her conclusions beyond the strain of rat with which an experiment had been performed. Given that moral philosophers want their conclusions to be widely, even universally, applicable, it seems helpful to test them empirically against the widest possible range of ways of life before making claims to representativity.

Serious bioethical engagement with disability issues should raise fundamental questions about the *kind of knowledge* that is needed to make moral decisions concerning people with different embodiments from our own, and the nature of the decisions that it is possible to make with the knowledge that can be obtained. These latter questions are epistemological rather than ethical. In this chapter I demonstrate why it is not ethically safe to trust commonality of moral background or ability to imagine the lives of others. I look at the suggestion that in order to do *ethical* work, bioethics needs to draw on a different pool of *epistemic* resources than has so far been the case. I argue that this is particularly true for bioethics' engagement with impairment and disability. For reasons that will become clear, I don't want to split apart the empirical and normative domains of bioethical inquiry. However, I give closer attention to what sort of normative claim can be made by empirical and experiential data in chapter 8. Here, I focus more on epistemic needs.

THE EMPIRICAL TURN WITHIN BIOETHICS

Although I've said bioethics is still a predominantly philosophical enterprise, it is also clear that in the last fifteen years or so it has taken a palpably empirical turn, driven in part by the social science critique of it (DeVries and Subedi 1998; Nelson 2000b; Zussman 2000; Turner 2004; Holm and Jonas 2004; Sugarman 2004; DeVries et al. 2007). In a study published in 2006, Borry et al. surveyed nine peer-reviewed journals in bioethics to estimate the proportion of published studies using some kind of empirical methodology. They reported a rise from 5.4 percent in 1990 to 15.4 percent in 2003, with around two-thirds being quantitative and one-third qualitative studies, and the highest proportion published in journals of nursing and medical and clinical ethics. The rising interest in empirical approaches has unsettled the methodological consensus in bioethics, and prompted lively ongoing debate about the relationship between descriptive/empirical and prescriptive/normative knowledge, and about the most appropriate methodologies for empirical bioethical research. The central theoretical problem here is how to relate descriptive information about actual moral orders to the normative statements ethics is supposed to make, a version of the long-standing philosophical debate about the nature of facts and values in different disciplines. Empirical study is held to deal in facts, while ethics as normally understood deals prescriptively in values and norms; but ethics still must have some grounding in fact, if the values and norms it prescribes are to have any meaning for the practices of the real world.

Empirical ethics and bioethics, by definition, are distinguished by their use of empirical methods at some point in the bioethical enterprise.[2] They share the view that in a situation of bioethical interest, a knowledge of people's actual behavior and thinking is useful for analyzing it ethically, devising and monitoring appropriate interventions, or formulating good policy. Most empirical ethicists favor standard social science methodologies,[3] including ethnography (Fox and Swazey 1992; Anspach 1993; Becker 2000; Rapp 2000), interviews and questionnaires (Scully et al. 2004, 2007), and sometimes more phenomenological or narrative resources. The most minimal view is one in which bioethics has an empirical arm whose job it is to identify the issues that need normative attention (Brody 1993). Bioethics then considers those problems and returns them, sorted, to the practitioners' domain. Beyond this point, approaches to empirical ethics diversify, and various attempts have been made to classify them by aim, methodology, or philosophical basis. Molewijk et al. (2004) identify five separate ways of using empirical data in ethics, four "traditional" and one "integrated." The traditional uses are distinguished according to whether final authority lies in moral theory or in the empirically observed social practice. In these terms, *prescriptive applied ethicists* and *theorists* both locate ultimate authority in moral theory. The function of empirical investigation is to support the application of theory to real life by "scooping up facts" (Nelson 2000b, 13) about everyday moral practices, which are then handed over to ethics for evaluative judgment against moral theory, or by monitoring the real-life consequences of a clinical or policy decision which can be used to inform a consequentialist evaluation. *Particularists,* on the other hand, claim to dissociate the morality of a social practice from moral theory. This approach has greater appeal to the more social science–inclined bioethicists than it does to philosophers, and it also leaves itself open to accusations of out-and-out moral relativism (Gewirth 1988), or of not being "ethics" at all. *Critical applied ethicists* in this typology see the relationship between moral theory and empirical knowledge as interactive, and they hold back from deciding a priori whether moral theory on the one hand or social practice on the other has final moral authority. Moral theory becomes "just one way to reflect on a social practice" (Molewijk et al. 2004, 56), and a critical approach can be brought to examine the background assumptions of a moral theory and see whether in reality they hold up in the situations they are supposed to (Musschenga 1999).

Using empirical data in ethics in these ways retains a traditional belief, weakest in the case of critical applied ethics, in the separation of empirical and normative disciplines. In contrast, what has been described as *integrated empirical ethics* claims distinction in seeing the empirical and the normative as mutually constitutive. Proponents of this approach agree with many contemporary theorists of knowledge that supposedly value-neutral, empirical disciplines are inevitably underpinned by discipline-specific epistemic biases, while moral theory in its turn is always backgrounded by historically and culturally specific empirical assumptions. This makes "collecting and classifying empirical data . . . in itself a normative process" (Molewijk et al. 2004, 61).

Based on published work, however, it is hard to see a real difference between critical applied ethics and integrated empirical ethics, except in that the studies published under the heading of integrated empirical ethics have so far concerned specific practices in clinical settings and have had the overtly normative goal of improving that practice (van der Scheer and Widdershoven 2004; Stiggelbout et al. 2004; Ebbesen and Pedersen 2007; for comparison see Nikku and Eriksson 2006). The epistemological stance also bears a strong resemblance to the *critical bioethics* introduced by some sociological bioethicists (Haimes 2002; Hedgecoe 2004) and to the feminist account I outline later. Hedgecoe describes critical bioethics as an approach that is "politely sceptical," involving "critical self-reflection on the nature of bioethics and the decisions it supports" (Hedgecoe 2004, 134). It uses social science methods and research, but aims to judge ethical situations and decisions as well as document them.

Bioethics done in the empirical mode may reveal discrepancies between what moral philosophers believe, what variously situated other people believe, and what moral philosophers think other people believe. For example, there is empirical work investigating what laypeople think is fair that suggests that participants' ideas are not in line with a Rawlsian theory of distributive justice (Miller 1992). Similarly, our study of researchers, clinicians, and candidate patients for somatic gene therapies showed that in practice, patients often had very different opinions about net harm or benefit than did physicians (Scully et al. 2004). As yet, however, there are virtually no examples of avowedly empirical work in bioethics done with the aim of getting information relevant to disability. Tyson and Stoll (2003) and Major-Kincade et al. (2001) have looked at decisions to treat or withhold treatment from premature infants with severe impairments. These studies are described as "evidence-based ethics," and like a lot of work under this heading, they make unexamined assumptions about what constitutes relevant evidence, what constitutes benefit and cost, how these factors should be weighed up, and who among all the participating actors should contribute to the weighing up and when—all of which severely compromise the claim to involve genuinely ethical reflection. There are more examples of sociological or ethnographic studies of disability that were not performed with normative intent, but which have nevertheless been used for bioethical reflection. For example, bioethicists, including me, have drawn on studies of hearing-impaired people's attitudes toward genetic testing (Middleton et al. 1998, 2001; Stern et al. 2002) in the ethical discussion of these technologies.

Purpose-built, empirically based bioethical studies of disability face a number of obstacles. One problem that is common to all such endeavors is that the research must be multi- or interdisciplinary, since few bioethicists are adequately trained in empirical methods, and vice versa. Interdisciplinarity presents its own epistemic and practical challenges. Further, the topic of disability presents a unique set of methodological barriers. First is the need to clarify who, exactly, is the subject of research. The previous chapter emphasized the difficulty both researchers and activists have in agreeing on a definition of disability or impairment, and this means that, at worst, researchers risk studying a group of people who others will contest are not "really" disabled, or are not properly representative of disabled people.

A second barrier is the difficulty of gaining access to disabled people. Most empirical bioethics research is carried out in healthcare settings, usually involving healthcare personnel and sometimes patients, relatives, or carers. But the majority of disabled people are not ill, and in most cases have no more contact with healthcare services than anyone else. The disabled people who *are* accessible via healthcare services will tend to be the most severely impaired and living in special care, or those who are in rehabilitation following illness or accident, or those who have multiple health problems. These constitute only a minority of the disabled population. In two projects on genetic illness and ethical decisions (Scully et al. 2004, 2007), our group at the University of Basel found that the disabled people we wanted to interview, who were simply getting on with their lives with little or no medical contact, did not belong to the self-help or political advocacy groups we were in touch with, or read the magazines or websites dedicated to their impairment where we placed advertisements. So if researchers are interested in the moral beliefs and attitudes of "ordinary" disabled people, recruiting them for study can demand considerable ingenuity.

And once identified, it may turn out that disabled people are less than enthusiastic about participating in an ethical study anyway. Many will have had enough of being poked, prodded, and stared at in clinics and elsewhere, and they may assume this is what ethics research involves too. In Germany and Switzerland particularly, we found a hostility to "being scientifically investigated" that could be traced back to a taken-for-granted link between bioethics and eugenics. In our study of somatic gene therapy, for example, we were told by one gatekeeper of a German impairment group that it was pointless trying to persuade any of its members to be interviewed. People with that impairment had suffered notably under the eugenic practices of the Third Reich, and since bioethics today was assumed to be similarly in favor of eugenics, all bioethicists were damned by association. It can take time and patience to gain potential participants' trust; in the process, researchers are confronted with dilemmas about exploitation of participants that are familiar from feminist social science methodology (see, for example, Oakley 1981). Finally, it needs to be recognized (which is sometimes hard to do when fully immersed in research) that most people, disabled or not, really have very little motivation to take part in empirical ethical research. Such research is generally performed *on* them rather than *with* them; there is probably no benefit to them as individuals or as a group; they may have ample present and historical reasons to fear that it will be actively harmful; and most ethics committees recommend that they not even be paid for their trouble.

MORAL UNDERSTANDINGS

The sociological studies of the last decade or so have expanded the scope of the information we have about, and sometimes changed our view of, well-trodden bioethical issues. But empirical study does not a priori challenge the epistemological foundations on which the standard procedures of bioethical inquiry have been built. The classical epistemology of moral philosophy focuses on *individuals* acquiring and justifying reliable (true) moral knowledge. Bioethics thereby inherits an epistemic norm of a single subject in conscious pursuit of the knowledge (medical facts, information on actions and outcomes) that she needs to make ethically sound decisions. For such an epistemic subject the central concerns are to do with acquiring information, being sure of its factual accuracy, and avoiding biases in information provision and interpretation.

The social epistemologies favored by many feminist and other nonmainstream ethical approaches turn away from the individual, and thereby spotlight different concerns about the knowledge held by moral agents. Thus, feminist epistemologies have observed that gendered patterns of social advantage end up in similarly gendered distributions of epistemic authority. Following on from this, the feminist critique has been able to ask whether allocation of epistemic authority tracks with other, nongendered forms of social positioning as well.

A key theoretical contribution to feminist moral epistemology, Margaret Urban Walker's *Moral Understandings* (1998) starts from the premise that the choice of any one ethical theory to address a problem is made against a background of a prior decision about what constitutes moral evaluation. In practice, this prior decision is actually a given, since the underlying idea of how academic moral inquiry should be conducted is rarely challenged. Conventional moral philosophical analysis, according to Walker, operates within a *theoretical-juridical* template that takes a particular view of moral theory "as a compact, propositionally codifiable, impersonally action-guiding code within an agent, or as a compact set of law-like propositions that 'explain' the moral behavior of a well-formed moral agent" (Walker 1998, 7–8). Ethical inquiries within this theoretical-juridical template are characteristically individualist but also impersonal, disembodied, and rationalist. Because they view ethical knowledge as occupying a special epistemological domain of its own, separate from other kinds of knowledge, adherents to the theoretical-juridical model consider physical, social, material, emotional, and similar nonmoral data as peripheral to the making of moral judgments. The worldly particularities of the people concerned and the settings they inhabit are irrelevant to producing the universal action-guiding codes that are the desired end.

It can be argued that this is an unkind caricature of real moral philosophy, conjured up for the rhetorical purpose of shooting it down. As the earlier discussion showed, bioethics' empirical turn is indicative of a growing acceptance of contextuality and greater questioning of the epistemological uniqueness of moral knowledge. Still, we need to keep in mind that empirical work remains a minority enthusiasm in bioethics. (If 15 percent of published bioethics papers in 2003 were empirical, that means 85 percent weren't.) And Walker's real point is not that this is how all ethical or bioethical inquiry is done, but that it remains the underlying ideal for how it *should* be done. She considers it to be both an inadequate template for conducting ethical inquiry, and an inaccurate picture of how it actually is conducted. Her proposed alternative, by now well known in feminist ethics, rejects a picture of moral life as a project pursued by an individual and involving a series of more or less rational choices. Instead she offers a picture of morality as a collaborative social practice through which people acknowledge and construct relationships, responsibilities, and commitments. This *expressive-collaborative* model represents moral life as an interpersonal enterprise, and so shifts the focus of ethical attention away from the generation of action guides and onto the values and practices that, a long way down the line, give rise to articulated moral principles. Everyday morality does involve the making of judgments and choices, but traditional moral philosophy spends a disproportionate amount of time on these activities. Just as much attention should be directed to the other activities of perception, description, interpretation, communication, narration, explanation, defense, response, and so on that constitute the bulk of everyday moral life.

Walker contends that moral behavior takes place against backgrounds of implicit knowledge that "constrain and make intelligible" the interactions between people within a community. Background moral understandings are conveyed to us by the communities in which we live. They include stories about good lives, and accounts of precedent that indicate the sorts of practices and choices that the community expects, and so they certainly do guide actions. But beyond that, they also provide the vocabulary for narrating and justifying our actions. They indicate the appropriate roles and institutions through which aspects of moral life are expressed and instruct on common moral practices such as assigning blame, demanding punishment, and accepting or avoiding responsibility. Moral understandings like these are not articulated in the codified form that the theoretical-juridical model recognizes. They have to be absorbed from the practices and discourses through which people make sense of events and relationships (Walker 1998, 10). Because moral theories and normative judgments are meaningful to people as they are implemented as practices, academic ethical analysis requires a sound knowledge of those practices in order to make sense of the theories and judgments being enacted. Academic ethics then reflects on how people express moral identity and agency through particular attempts to live in what they understand as good ways, within the contingent possibilities and limitations of those lives.

By redirecting ethical attention toward social contexts, the expressive-collaborative model presses us to take a more *critical* view of the nature of the moral knowledge being held up as authoritative. People come to occupy differing social positions that influence the opportunities made available or the obligations assigned to them, and as a result they are likely to be confronted with different moral issues; this is not controversial. A more contentious suggestion is that moral subjects in different social positions experience similar moral issues differently, because they have different reserves of economic, social, and cultural capital to draw on, and because they will differ in their perception and weighing up of the situation's parameters

(Walker 1998, 50). A socially marginalized woman carrying a fetus with an impairment, for example, may come to a different conclusion about the morality of terminating her pregnancy than a more affluent, socially secure woman would,[4] and this may be quite reasonably based on the different costs and risks to which women in the two social positions are exposed.

Walker is making two different but related points about moral episte-mology. The first is that moral knowledge is no longer epistemologically special territory. If moral understandings are generated out of the concrete circumstances of communities and the relationships of their members (Walker 1998, 111–13), then in order to comprehend them, and then to evaluate them, we need a grasp of "the specific ways goods and selves are understood in continuing and evolving traditions within communities" (Walker 1998, 19). A naturalized moral epistemology is interested in deter-mining how to reach the point where we can reasonably claim to know *enough* about particular situations and the people who encounter them to assess them ethically. Feminists criticize prefeminist moral philosophy for taking for granted that those conditions of inquiry are present, for assum-ing that "we" (those of us reflecting on a moral problem, or evaluating other people's solutions to it) are already familiar enough with these situa-tions and persons to make those kinds of moral judgments. That epistemo-logical confidence goes hand in hand with the belief that people, or per-haps just people who matter, do not vary much in terms of the moral terrain they occupy. If that's true, the chances are high that others will agree with the way I frame a given situation, weigh up morally salient features of it, and carry my argument through to a conclusion. But if this is not true— if it isn't the case that moral understanding is very similar between agents— then ethics must systematically analyze the "actual moral arrangements" of what people in the situations of interest really do, and what reasons can be found for those acts and choices. Walker sees generating such an "empiri-cally saturated" analysis as ethics' most neglected task, joining Annette Baier and other feminist ethicists who have called for philosophy to collaborate with empirical social disciplines to find out what moral lives entail (Baier 1985, 224).

The second, harder point about moral epistemology is that the under-standings up for critical scrutiny always include our own. Theories of knowl-edge that consider social and historical position as significant must conclude that any ethical reflection is inescapably along a specific line of sight, deter-mined, among other things, by the identity of the knower. It is fair to say that until very recently, the profession of moral philosophy was staffed by a so-cially limited subgroup of people: overwhelmingly male, affluent enough to be educated, mostly white and from Judeo-Christian cultural backgrounds, and mostly not disabled except by the common impairments of age. The taken-for-granted forms of knowledge in moral philosophy, and by extension bioethics, are epistemically skewed to reflect the circumstances of this statistically quite anomalous group of knowers.

If we take this diagnosis seriously, bioethicists operate under a requirement for constant self-scrutiny of facts taken for granted and values assumed to be shared. Unlike a straightforwardly empirical bioethics that sees it as useful and necessary to investigate the way that "ordinary people" go about making moral judgments, with the aim of seeing how they compare with the normative judgments of moral philosophy, an expressive-collaborative view of moral understandings does not separate lay knowledge from its academic version. As bioethicists we might be interested in the epistemic and ethical positions of a group whose moral reasoning we want to understand—say, members of the Deaf community who reject cochlear implants, or parents who want financial support to carers of disabled children to take priority over funding for research to prevent the disabling condition. We can aim to produce critical accounts of what these epistemic communities hold to be *true knowledge* and what their moral communities think of as *good lives*. We might try to give unbiased and accurate descriptions of ethically interesting situations, but we cannot make any claim for them as objective in the sense of Nagel's "view from nowhere" (1989). What we can do is apply the same critical stance to our own epistemic community of bioethicists. Some of the self-critique can be provided by other disciplines focusing on the cultural, economic, and political contexts that shape bioethicists' own lines of sight (DeVries 2002; Haimes 2002). This form of scrutiny contributes to what Sandra Harding and other feminist standpoint epistemologists have dubbed *strong objectivity* (Harding 1991, 1993; Hartsock 1987), that is, an objectivity that is not grounded in a (probably doomed) search for epistemic neutrality, but which through collecting and critiquing a diversity of viewpoints provides the resources for *better*, if not complete or unchallengeable, knowledge.

Although Walker wants to redress what she sees as an imbalance by encouraging moral philosophy to shoulder a greater "descriptive and empirical burden," it is important to be clear that the expressive-collaborative model does not see the tasks of ethics as ending with the investigation of forms of moral life. Taking what is now known about the moral understandings embedded in those lives, ethics then has to critically reflect on them, with the aim of seeing how normative they can be.

MORAL UNDERSTANDINGS OF/IN DISABILITY

This twofold modified view, first of how moral lives are constituted, and second of the task of ethical analysis, has radical implications for bioethics' engagement with disability. First, a "descriptive and empirical" bioethics of disability depends on an expanded program of moral inquiry into the lives of disabled people and those associated with them, involving sociological, historical, ethnographic, psychological, political, and other forms of empirical research. We want to improve our empirical grounding in aspects of those lives that are of bioethical relevance—the processes of decision making about impaired infants in neonatal care units, as one example. And since comprehending the moral understandings of different communities involves knowing "what it is like to live out the arrangements that embody the understandings, how it feels and seems to live them" (Walker 2002, 181), bioethical inquiry also needs to elicit the idiographic, phenomenological accounts of disabled people.

Empirical and phenomenological information helps fill out our factual knowledge of situations where impairment is an issue. Effective engagement, though, requires something more than improving our empirical grounding. Bioethical analysis should have at least an inkling of how and why particular groups of people, disabled or nondisabled, adopt the solutions or range of solutions they do. Moreover, if communities arrive at shared moral understandings after the negotiation of evidence and interpretation, then there are pertinent questions to be asked about who has or is given the power to take part in those negotiations. The kind of critical moral epistemology I have been describing pays closer attention to the procedures and patterns of dominance that enable the perspectives of nondisabled people to take precedence over those of disabled people, or particular types of impairment over other types. It encourages questions about how social and political structures give some people more voice than others, for instance, and asks whether and in what ways the resulting allocation of epistemic authority is unjust.

Miranda Fricker (2007) has identified two distinct forms of epistemic injustice that follow the marginalization of social groups. One, which is relevant to the discussion of narrative identity I take up in chapter 6, she calls *hermeneutical injustice*. She defines this as "having some significant area of one's social experience obscured from collective understanding owing to a structural prejudice in the collective hermeneutical resource" (Fricker 2006, 100). In other words, the marginalization of social groups extends to the neglect or suppression of concepts and narratives that would enable them and others to make sense of their particular experience. While sexuality, for example, is a significant area for most people in the discourse of contemporary life, the sexuality of disabled people is rarely discussed with the same openness. As a result, many disabled people reach adulthood without having access to appropriate information and vocabulary about sexuality or sexual ethics, and without the opportunity to develop *the idea* of a sexual life within the particular parameters of their impairment (Shakespeare et al. 1996, 22–29).

Fricker distinguishes this from a second form of epistemic injustice, *testimonial injustice*, in which prejudice against a group results in its members' being given less credibility than they would otherwise enjoy. Testimonial injustice, in the form of having one's own account dismissed, is commonplace in the interactions between disabled and nondisabled people. Of course, there are impairments that genuinely do compromise a person's ability to understand events and experiences.[5] Fricker's point, though, refers to an undifferentiated response to disabled people, irrespective of the nature of the impairment. Later on in this chapter I discuss the paradox that disabled people may report a quality of life almost equivalent to that reported by nondisabled people, and significantly higher than that imagined by nondisabled people. When this paradox is brought to their attention, nondisabled commentators are likely to respond with versions of "she would say that, wouldn't she," explaining that newly disabled people are using denial to avoid mental distress, and long-term disabled people are unable to make unbiased appraisals of their lives because they don't know any better. In my experience, what *doesn't* happen is that the nondisabled observer agrees that disabled people might in fact be best placed to know how satisfactory their own lives are. In this response, the accounts of disabled people are dismissed because they are assumed to be inherently untrustworthy and possibly self-serving, in a way that those of nondisabled people are not. In the disability world there are many similar stories of the denial of epistemic authority, and its consequences, ranging from the tragic (discounting the evidence of sexually abused disabled children: see Shakespeare et al. 1996, 135–45; Hardiker 1994, 262) to the merely infuriating: for many years, the BBC's flagship disability program was called *Does He Take Sugar?* in honor of a paradigmatic example.

MORAL COMMUNITIES

Walker suggests that moral understandings are shared in moral communities. But what constitutes a moral community? It is not moral unanimity. Sharing a moral understanding does not imply that everyone in the community agrees with it or is united on how best to live it out in everyday institutions. A moral understanding is held in common when the group members recognize that it has "force in defining responsibilities and prerogatives" (Walker 1998, 7): they acknowledge it as meaningful, if not necessarily right. It seems likely that the extent to which moral communities are coterminous with other community or group identities varies and needs to be determined on a case-by-case basis. It would also be a mistake to assume that all levels of moral understanding are shared within a moral community. A foundational conviction that there *are* morally better and worse ways in which to live might be shared with all other human beings, and we might want to go further to suggest that some injunctions on modes of conduct are common to all communities, but the degree of commonality decreases the more specific the moral prescriptions become.

The proposition that disabled people form a moral community runs into the problems I discussed in chapter 2. Given the diversity of impairments and the difficulty of defining impairment or disability, it is not immediately obvious what the idea of a "community" of disabled people would mean in terms of moral understanding. Minimal moral understandings are likely to be common to everyone, disabled or not. Some others may be shared by all disabled people by virtue of their impairment, through the experience of oppression (according to the strong social model), or encountering blocks in sociocultural interactions (in other social-relational models), or deviating from a biological norm (in a medicalized model). Some others may be shared by people with particular types of impairment, perhaps common to those with mobility impairments but not to others who have visual impairments. Yet other moral communities might be formed through the intersections of impairment with other kinds of identity, as suggested by recent work in disability studies exploring the lives of disabled women, or disabled members of ethnic or sexual minorities (Fine and Asch 1988; Wendell 1996; Ahmad 2000; Hernandez 2005; Whitney 2006), which might mean that disabled women will tend to agree on certain moral issues that disabled men do not. And so on.

Walker's use of moral communities has been accused of falling into, or at least veering dangerously toward, the trap of parochialism (Card 2002, 151). It risks weakening any sense of moral solidarity with those with whom we *don't* claim a common understanding. In response, it helps to remember here that the "communities" in question are more analytic than they are ontological. In reality, their boundaries are permeable, and they are not mutually exclusive. The accusation of parochialism loses its force once it is recognized that real social groupings are always fragmented, so that any individual with impairment will inevitably have membership of several interlocking, overlapping communities. Because of this, although moral understandings develop out of negotiations within groups, they are at the same time devised with one eye on commitments elsewhere. In practice, both the richness and difficulties of moral life are a result of interplay between moral communities. It feels to me, for instance, that my internalized moral terrain has been built up from, variously, membership in the cultural community of the post-Enlightenment West, the national community of the English, the working-class and immigrant Asian culture I grew up in and the middle-class academic world I'm now part of, the religious community I chose to join, and a mixed chosen/unchosen solidarity with hearing-impaired and other disabled people. Personal observation makes me realize that precisely which associated moral understanding is mobilized depends strongly on what the moral issue is; whether its effects are direct or, conversely, whether I am reflecting on it as part of my professional obligations; and whose company I am in (that is, which community I feel most part of) at the time.

Theoretical reflection around questions of moral community and identity in bioethical contexts has so far been sparse: "the" moral community has been assumed to be unitary. Feminist bioethics has taken the lead here in theorizing around gender and other social identities. Much classic feminist bioethical work asks whether, and if so in what ways and through which processes, women experience events differently from men; and then how women's views are inserted into or excluded from mainstream medical and ethical discourse (see, for example, Holmes and Purdy 1992; Sherwin 1992; Little 1996; Sherwin et al. 1998; Rawlinson 2001; Tong et al. 2004). Analogous work has begun for ethnic, cultural, or sexual orientation identities. But disability's peculiarities of diversity, definition, and possible intrinsic disadvantage make it unlike gender or any of the other organizational categories, and that means it presents distinctive challenges to theories of social-moral epistemology.

LIMITS TO MORAL IMAGINATION

Bioethics' involvement with disability has predominantly concerned moral judgments about the quality of life. These judgments assess what it is like to live with an impairment and decide whether, according to that assessment, further steps are morally permissible or not. Making moral judgments about the quality of another life requires at least (1) an adequate grasp of what the features of that life are; (2) agreement about which of these are relevant to making that assessment, that is, a background theory about what constitutes "quality" in a life; and (3) a way of measuring those relevant features against some kind of standard. Phenotypic variation raises difficulties at all of these points: (1) it is questionable whether most people, even those of us who for professional or personal reasons have to make judgments about the lives of others, have an adequate grasp of the lives of people with impairments; (2) without this knowledge, we cannot know for sure which are the relevant features, or whether disabled people find all or some of the same features as relevant as nondisabled people do; (3) as the criteria for evaluation are set, by and large, by nondisabled people and evaluated with reference to their own experience, there is a risk that the criteria, or their weighting, or both, will be inappropriate to the lived experience of impairment.

Bioethics tends to assume that these difficulties can be overcome by the exercise of moral imagination. I suggested earlier that classical moral theory works "with a picture of knowledge for which right perception is 'alike' in moral agents, who therefore readily 'put themselves in someone else's shoes'" (Code 2002, 158). By imaginatively "putting ourselves in someone else's shoes," it is argued, it is possible to understand the experiences and perspectives of those whose lives are quite different from our own. But high-profile controversies in bioethics indicate that there are barriers to imagining the quality of life of those whose bodily experiences differ substantially from one's own. An example is the case of Bree Walker, an American actor and broadcaster with the rare genetic condition of ectrodactyly, an anomaly in which fingers and sometimes toes show varying degrees of fusion. In 1994, when she had already given birth to one child who had inherited the condition and was pregnant with another, she took part in a radio phone-in program in which the presenter asked the audience, "Is it fair for Bree to have children [at all] knowing that she might pass ectrodactyly along to her children?" In the phone-in many participants argued that she was being irresponsible in bringing into the world a child with the same impairment as herself, because of the suffering and disadvantages he or she would experience. The intriguing thing about this incident is that the callers were apparently unable to recognize Walker's self-assessment that this phenotypic variation had not presented a major problem in her life. Even given that information, they could not imaginatively project beyond their conviction that ectrodactyly must inevitably hinder life achievement and satisfaction.

"Putting yourself in x's shoes" means trying to see things from the point of view of another whose situation and perspective appears very different from our own, or whose actions and judgments we find disturbing or incomprehensible. It suggests that we need to engage imaginatively with another's point of view in order to understand her. A number of moral and political philosophers over the centuries have taken up this idea, from Hume's claim that moral judgment requires an agent to counter his natural tendencies toward partiality by trying to find "a point of view common to him with others" (Hume 1968, 252), to those interpreters of Rawls's original position (Rawls 1971), including Kymlicka (2002), who think that the representatives behind the veil of ignorance have to divest themselves of knowledge of their own situation and imaginatively take up the situation of others. In the philosophy of mind, simulation theorists propose that understanding other people's thought processes involves simulating their mental states in our own minds.[6] By simulating or imaginatively recreating another person's thought processes, we assume that the other person's reasoning processes work along the same lines as ours, and if we have a baseline of knowledge about their beliefs and values we ought to be able to follow their thinking, even if we don't agree with them. In feminist philosophy, Maria Lugones refers to "playful 'world' travelling" to describe entering into the experiences of others as a way of identifying with them, "because by traveling to their 'world' we can understand what it is to be them and what it is to be ourselves in their eyes" (1990, 401).

But the evidence I've presented here suggests that there are greater limits to this than we might want to think. One difficulty with "putting oneself in another's shoes" is that there is more than one mode of imaginative projection, and these modes make different contributions to the expansion of moral competence. If I simply imagine myself in the other's situation, I enact the narrative that I imagine I would enact if it were me. In this kind of imaginative projection I am imagining not another person, but myself in a different setting, and I am drawing on my own experience. I imagine myself as unable to walk, for example, or with fused fingers. Everything else about me (character, interests, relationships, occupation, biases, and so on) remains the same: the single change is that I now use a wheelchair or have difficulty buying gloves. This kind of imagination lends itself best to perceiving the practical adjustments that would have to be made to accommodate the impairment. The more detailed the factual knowledge about the particular impairment, the more likely I will be able to anticipate, to some extent, what it would be like if I myself were in that situation. I might go so far as to borrow a wheelchair, or tape my fingers together, to make the imaginative engagement more vivid. The success of this version of imagining oneself as other depends on factors such as how well I really can anticipate my responses, how much information I have about the experience and how accurate the information is, and whether I have gone through anything analogous from which I can extrapolate more or less accurately (being temporarily unable to walk because of a broken leg, for example).

A second mode of imaginative projection involves going beyond imagining myself in the situation, and imagining myself *as* that other person.[7] Whether or not I can do this successfully depends additionally on how much I know and understand about the other person in terms of her character, history, interests, and emotional attitudes. Another requirement is sensitivity to the differences in gender, age, culture, religion, or class between me and the other person that might compromise my ability to extrapolate accurately from one to the other. Often, however, there will be too many aspects of the other into which I have no insight or which I do not share. Therefore, it is most likely that attempts at this kind of imaginative projection will involve a mixing of the other person's perspective with my own.

Theorists also propose a third kind of imagining oneself as other: empathetic imagining (Goldie 2000), in which our own perspectives are left behind and we genuinely adopt the other's thoughts, feelings, and emotions. This requires us unself-consciously to "inhabit" the other person's cognitive and emotional responses, and also her embodied modes of engagement with the world. Whether this is ever achievable in day-to-day life is, to my mind, doubtful, for the reasons given above. (It might conceivably be possible in some altered states of consciousness, or through some future technology that allows the transfer of mental states.)

Reflecting the concept of the mind as something like pure intelligence or rationality, moral imagination is conventionally considered to be a disembodied capacity. Catriona Mackenzie and I have argued elsewhere in more detail why we consider imagination to be fundamentally an embodied capacity of the mind (Mackenzie and Scully 2007), and why having/being a particular kind of body places real constraints on our capacities both to imagine ourselves otherwise and to imaginatively put ourselves in the place of others. In brief, imagination can be considered an embodied capacity because (1) there is no mental activity without a body (as far as anyone can prove); and (2) imaginative projection is dependent on personal experience (either of the same event, or something similar enough to form the basis for accurate imaginative projection), and therefore it is constrained by the particularities of the body because the experiences of persons are themselves dependent on the body.

The suggestion that embodied experience sets limits to the capacity for imaginative projection into another life is supported by more rigorous empirical work illustrating what some theorists describe as the central disability paradox (Albrecht and Devliger 1999). I mention earlier that studies assessing the quality of life after impairment (spinal cord injury, for example) sometimes indicate that "when asked about the quality of their own lives, disabled people report a quality only slightly lower than that reported by non-disabled people, and much higher than that projected by non-disabled people" (Amundsen 2005,103; see also Mehnert et al. 1990; Chase et al. 2000; Ville and Ravaud 2001; Horgan and MacLachlan 2004; Ubel et al. 2005). Some of the data even claim to show *no* change in overall life satisfaction (Stensman 1985; Cushman and Dijkers 1990). Most pertinent to the consideration of imaginative projection, even hospital and rehabilitation staff (who might be expected to have better than average insight into patients' lives) evaluated their patients' quality of life as lower than the patients themselves did (Gerhart et al. 1994; Cushman and Dijkers 1990; Riis et al. 2005).

Nondisabled commentators tend to explain the paradox by suggesting that newly disabled people make the best of a bad job: they use psychological mechanisms of adaptation, coping, and accommodation to avoid mental distress. In response, disability scholars have argued that "it is not clear that the difference between an individual's report of the quality of life she lives despite her limitations, and others' view of that life, is merely the difference between adaptation and nonadaptation" (Silvers 2005, 58). Jonathan Cole's study of the narratives of men with spinal cord injury identifies a wide range of responses to their new lives as paraplegic or tetraplegic. Among them are those who express something like Mike, one of the interviewees: "[Before the accident] I remember thinking clearly . . . that if it ever happened to me I could not stand it. I would want to kill myself. . . . But once it did happen to me, all the things I thought I would think and feel, I never felt at all" (Cole 2004, 211). The point I am trying to make is not that the impact of spinal cord injury on these men's lives is trivial, nor that they do not wish it had not happened, but rather that its effect is unpredictable within the parameters of prior experience.

These empirically observed discrepancies between reported and projected accounts of what it is like to live with an impairment point up how restricted is our ability to imagine the lives of others with very different phenotypic capacities. Up to a point, a critical and skeptical approach to statements that run counter to our own intuitions—like evaluations of postinjury quality of life—is appropriate. But we also need to be vigilant against the epistemic injustice identified by Fricker, or what James Lindemann Nelson has referred to as the epistemic "disability" conferred on those with a particular social identity, in this case that of a person with impairment (Nelson 2001).

To assume there can be no residuum of difference between ourselves and the other is empirically unsound. More than that, it is ultimately a dismissal of the other's identity as embodied, temporal, and placed. Indeed, Lugones' vision of "world-traveling" has been criticized for being "a new imagination of disembodiment: a dream of being *everywhere*" (Bordo 1990, 143) or everybody. These are the sorts of illusory epistemic practices that a critical moral epistemology should identify and correct for.

A central claim of this book is that the experiences of impairment and disability may contribute, in ways that are still largely unexplored, to differences in the perception and interpretation of morally relevant features of life. These differences may be enough to generate significantly different moral understandings of life events and choices. In this view, the central disability paradox is a result of situated differences in perception and understanding, and not necessarily of psychological defenses or epistemic inadequacy on the part of disabled people. When feminist and other theorists from marginal perspectives focus on the epistemic effects of being different, they are concerned mostly with the effects of social positioning: the difference that belonging to a particular social category makes. Standpoint epistemologies claim that there are cognitive and affective changes in the perception and interpretation of events that follow from being a member of a marginalized social group, not by virtue of social *position* as much as the associated social *practices* (Smith 1990), and that this gives an alternative or even privileged insight into the domains of life affected by subordinate social status (Hartsock 1987; Harding 1991, 1997; Haraway 1991; Stoetzler and Yuval-Davis 2002). Social identities are, clearly, often assigned as a result of the bodies people have or are. A social identity as a woman comes about when someone has a body that is phenotypically female, and feminists are interested in the epistemic, ethical, and other effects of that social positioning. But with the exception of some outstanding feminist phenomenological work (Young 2005; Bartky 1990, 2002; Fisher and Embree 2000), not much attention has yet been given to the *epistemic impact* of embodied difference more broadly, whether concentrating on biological difference, or differences in cultural representations, or in the available narratives of personal and collective identity.

In the following chapters I explore some theories that suggest how such differences might come about, and that therefore indicate methodological avenues for future research. Before doing so, it may be necessary to state explicitly that I do not put these particular explanations forward as the best or only ways to theorize the impact of impairment on moral life. In fact, I am not especially committed to the idea that phenotypic variation inevitably *does* make that kind of difference to moral perception and interpretation: on the available evidence it would be rash for anyone to make as strong a claim as that. My more modest commitments are to the ideas that phenotypic variation might make that kind of difference; that there has not been anything like enough empirical or experiential investigation into disability for us to know whether or not it does; and that there exist theoretical and methodological approaches that would at the very least provide us with a better insight into both the shared and the possibly divergent moral understandings of disabled and nondisabled people.

NOTES

1. Part of this chapter has appeared in Catriona Mackenzie and Jackie Leach Scully's "Moral Imagination, Disability and Embodiment," *Journal of Applied Philosophy* 24 (2007): 335–51.

2. Maya Goldenberg distinguishes empirical approaches to ethics from "evidence-based ethics," in part because she finds that the latter narrows the scope of the empirical data it uses to medical outcomes, excluding most forms of qualitative and social scientific evidence (Goldenberg 2005, 11). See also Borry et al. (2006).

3. A common weakness of discussions of empirical approaches to ethics is the tendency to minimize major methodological and philosophical differences between different forms of social science inquiry.

4. She would not necessarily and invariably come to a different conclusion, but she might.

5. This should not be taken as a global assessment either. Some people with learning disabilities perceive and interpret events very accurately indeed, and not all forms of mental illness affect a person's judgment severely, or all the time. But in both these cases, the nature of the impairment would make it legitimate to be, initially at least, more cautious; this would not be true for other kinds of impairment.

6. See, for example, Davies and Stone (1995).

7. Goldie (2000) refers to this as "in-the-other's-shoes-imagining."

4

Different by Choice?

Just beneath the surface, there's this deaf person. I'm not talking about hearing loss, I'm talking about a whole way of being. The real me is Deaf. If you want to know me, you've got to know that part of me.

—Hearing adult of deaf parents

INFAMOUS DEAF BABIES

Hearing-impaired people occupy a unique position in the disabled/ nondisabled taxonomy. While the majority of hearing and many hearing-impaired people consider audiological deafness a disability, an increasing number inside and outside the Deaf world argue that being deaf is more like being a member of a distinct social or ethnic group than it is like other physical impairments. At the extreme end of this continuum are culturally Deaf people who consider themselves to be members of a minority cultural group and not to have an impairment at all—at least not in the right contexts (Lane 1992; Jennifer Harris 1995). They may not feel they have much in common with other disabled people: Ladd and John write, "Labelling us as 'disabled' demonstrates a failure to understand that we are not disabled in any way within our own community. . . . Many disabled people see Deaf people as belonging, with them, outside the mainstream culture. We, on the other hand, see disabled people as 'hearing' people in that they use a different language to us" (Ladd and John 1991, 14–15).

The "Deaf community" claims its own language and its own distinctive culture, though there is also debate about what this really means, theoretically

and in practice (Jennifer Harris 1995; Corker 2002; Sparrow 2005). I take up
the question of disability culture and community again in chapter 7. For now,
let's take it that by the criteria of having a distinct language, unique practices,
some shared history, and specialized social organizations (like schools for the
deaf, Deaf social clubs, and nowadays online Deaf groups), it makes sense to
talk of a distinct Deaf culture or Deaf world. The way in which the Deaf community comes into being, however, also leads to unanticipated (for the outsider) complications. More than one author, for instance, suggests that it is
not necessary to be *deaf* in order to be Deaf: "While some degree of hearing
loss is necessary for a person to be ethnically Deaf, the loss of hearing per se
is not the critical variable. Many individuals have only a minor hearing impairment in audiological terms but still are recognized as Deaf persons according to social and cultural criteria. On the other hand, some people with
very profound hearing losses are not considered to be Deaf according to those
same criteria" (Johnson and Erting 1982, 234).

Although the evidence suggests that the majority of culturally Deaf people express no preference for having either deaf or hearing children (Stern
et al. 2002; Middleton et al. 2001), there are some who do. It was a case in
which such a preference was acted on that caused a flurry of media attention in early 2002, and the story has provided fuel for bioethical discussion ever since (Anstey 2002; Levy 2002a; Savulescu 2002; Häyri 2004;
Johnston 2005; Parker 2007).[1] A lesbian couple from Washington, D.C.,
Sharon Duchesneau and Candace McCullough, wanted to have a child by
donor insemination. Both had a congenital and probably genetic hearing
impairment, and they chose to increase their chances of having a deaf
child by using sperm from a donor who also had a heritable form of deafness. Despite what has been stated in some popular accounts—and it is
important to stress this—Duchesneau and McCullough did not reject the
idea of having a hearing child. What they did was clearly express a *preference* for a hearing-impaired one, saying that while any child would be a
gift, a deaf one would be "a special gift." Their problem was that commer-
cial sperm banks do not use donors with known heritable disease or impairment, and that includes hearing impairment. As a result the couple
eventually came to a private arrangement with a male friend with genetic
deafness, resulting so far in the birth of two children, both of them hearing impaired (Mundy 2002).

Responses to the women's decision were markedly polarized. Most common was disapproval: not because of their decision to have a child, but because they tried to up the chances of its having a hearing impairment.[2] Even
in commentaries that were mainly supportive there was an underlying sense
of incomprehension that anyone should want to do this. For example, Liza
Mundy, a sympathetic journalist who wrote the major feature on Duchesneau and McCullough in the *Washington Post*, nevertheless said that it might

be seen as "a shocking undertaking" (Mundy 2002). Meanwhile, and in stark contrast, some advocates for the Deaf community (both Deaf and hearing) strongly defended the couple's right not only to have a child but to choose the *kind* of child they wanted to have.

Some time later, it was reported from Australia that a hearing-impaired Melbourne couple planned to use preimplantation genetic diagnosis (PGD) to screen their embryos and thereby *ensure* (not, like Duchesneau and McCullough, merely increase their chances) that they would have a child with normal hearing. In marked contrast to the earlier case, there was virtually no ethical debate about the actions of these parents. The lack of any demand for justification here suggests that most people felt the choice in this case to be uncontentiously right. Interestingly, the newspaper report *did* mention that because the legal use of PGD in Australia is restricted to preventing the transmission of genetic disease, it was necessary for the local regulatory body, the Infertility Treatment Authority, to decide on the legitimacy of the request because "we have to ask if deafness is a disease. . . . Some people would say deafness is a disease. Others would say it was an unfortunate condition" (Riley 2002). But there was no hint of the position taken by some Deaf people, that it is neither of these but instead a different way of being in the world.

In the debate around the Duchesneau-McCullough decision, arguments both in opposition and support were almost exclusively based on concepts of parental (and sometimes societal) rights and obligations. First, there were those who argued that a child has a right not to be harmed and therefore parents have a concomitant obligation not to harm her. In this case, the harm consists in condemning the child to a disability that could have been avoided.[3] A more elaborate version of this draws on Joel Feinberg's notion that a child has a right to have "future options kept open until he [*sic*] is a fully formed self-determining adult capable of deciding among them" (Feinberg 1992, 77). In a well-known article on using genetic testing to implement parental desires, dating from before the Duchesneau-McCullough story, Dena Davis locates the central moral problem in the damage being done to this right. Davis holds that parents are acting unethically if they make genetic selections that reduce the range of futures open to their children. She argues that a disability, such as being hearing impaired, will necessarily narrow the range of choices that could otherwise be available to the child as she grows up. Davis carefully avoids being drawn into a discussion of whether being deaf is itself a harm. She instead concentrates on what she identifies as parental disregard for this child's right, in that the deliberate choice of impairment condemns the child "forever to a narrow group of people and a limited choice of careers" (Davis 1997, 14).[4] The disregard is manifest by (1) forcing the child irreversibly into the parental idea of what constitutes a good life, which Davis emphasizes is especially problematic where this is not a notion of the good life that is generally held, or (2) in the particular case of hearing impairment, being treated solely as a means to the end of perpetuating Deaf culture. Davis believes that, in a liberal state, having a diversity of communities (including the Deaf community) generally *increases* autonomy because it increases the number of ways in which people may elect to live. However, this benefit can exist only if individuals are in fact free to choose which community they want to be part of, and Davis thinks that certain parental choices—like selecting for hearing impairment, or perhaps even choosing not to select against it—will reduce or eliminate that freedom. And where the demands of the group conflict with the right of the individual to (be able to) make such life choices, the liberal state must, Davis believes, support the ethical priority of the individual.[5]

Davis' article has been critiqued on a number of points. Crucially, the intuitively attractive concept of an "open future" is less solid than it first appears. Given that all parents make decisions about the form and content of a child's life from the moment it is born (and often before), including the education it gets and the company it keeps, *any* child's future must be seen as significantly constrained by the decisions of its parents. These choices mean that at no point do children have what could feasibly be called "open futures" because options are already closed off. In everyday life we don't normally take exception to this: we understand that no child can survive, let alone flourish, in the absence of a familial and social framework that guides its development and, in doing so, inevitably restricts some choices and behaviors. The discussion in the bioethical literature focuses on distinguishing which kinds of parental choices sustain or, even better, enhance a child's future capacity to make responsible and autonomous life choices (Buchanan et al. 2000; Savulescu 2001, 2007).

Davis and others who use this argument, however, may fail to be sufficiently critical of their background assumptions about the nature of autonomous choices or good lives. Davis, for example, says at one point that having parents choose to ensure their children are achondroplasic is acceptable because restricted growth does not constrain futures as much as hearing impairment does (Davis 2001, 66). But aside from her own opinion she does not provide any empirical or other evidence to back this up, and other observers—deaf, achondroplasic, or neither of these—might disagree with her judgment. Relying on a liberal paradigm in which autonomous choice per se has high value, these commentators often imply that it is the sheer number of possible open futures that matters. Eric Schmidt says that parents who, given the choice, opt for hearing "allow their child to have many experiences she would not otherwise have had. It would limit their child from having a few experiences, such as becoming fully fluent in sign language or becoming part of the Deaf culture . . . [b]ut the added possible experiences would significantly outnumber the precluded possible experiences" (Schmidt 2007, 195). But this seems to me to give an odd picture of what we ought to consider important here, which is surely more a matter of what particular futures contain for the life of the child: the "mere multiplication of opportunities does not increase our chances of leading a meaningful or worthwhile life" (Sparrow 2005, 143).

Another difficulty of these arguments is that they may use an oversimplified model of what a community is and how it functions. Communities are treated as things that an individual can simply decide to leave or to join (see the discussion in Corker 1998b, 21–25). But the evidence of sociology and social psychology suggests that community identifications are not so easily manipulated. How easily people migrate from one culture to another depends on factors such as language abilities; the strength of community ties and the extent to which they are identity constituting; the relative esteem in which cultures are held; the circumstances under which a community accepts an incomer; and many others. Hence cultural and social groups are not items of clothing to be swapped at will. "You can take the girl out of X but you can't take X out of the girl," where X is any social grouping from "Southall" to "the chorus," makes an old but valid point.

Whether for or against the Duchesneau-McCullough choice, all these ethical analyses focus on rights and the preservation of individual (the child's) autonomy. In doing so, however, they sidestep the question of why the rightness or wrongness of the decision seemed so *obvious* to the various agents and commentators. There were those, probably the majority, for whom willingly opting for a child with a hearing impairment was unquestionably a harm. And there were those, predominantly but not solely from the Deaf community or disability activist groups, for whom hearing impairment was either not a disadvantage, or not enough of a disadvantage to make this parental choice reprehensible. The liberal, rights-based framework that most commentaries used is capable of analyzing whether or not Duchesneau and McCullough were expressing a legitimate preference, in terms of particular ideas about the limits to parental rights over their children, but does not take up the question of why the couple thought that it *was* a legitimate preference while others vehemently disagreed. Almost certainly, Duchesneau and McCullough did not set out from the premise that they should "exercise a right" to have whatever kind of child they felt like. Their preference must have seemed to them both intuitively correct and rationally justifiable. Even sympathetic commentators found that hard to take; meanwhile, some Deaf activists struggled to grasp what the opponents' problem was. And yet one of the most striking features of the whole debate was the lack of interest in finding out what these entrenched normative convictions were based on.

If moral perspectives are shaped by the experience of disabled embodiment, then mutual incomprehension can arise because the lived experiences of hearing-impaired and unimpaired persons are not as straightforwardly interchangeable as a decontextualized analysis would have it. They are not the same lives, plus or minus sound. A decontextualized analytic approach falls in line with traditional approaches to moral philosophy, according to which moral agents are pretty much interchangeable, and knowing the ethically correct way forward in any given situation should not require more than an outline knowledge of doer and done-to, or the circumstances in which it all takes place. But we know that real moral agents don't (can't) behave like this. Traditional ethical theories knowingly present an idealized version of human behavior that reflects the assumptions that moral agents can be isolated from their community bonds and from their corporeality. Real moral agents are embodied, however, and embodiment—as male or female, hearing or deaf—is a biological and material particularity that informs social relationships and physical capacities. Together, embodied and social interactions build a moral terrain within which certain judgments are justifiable. A different embodiment, and/or different social interactions, will generate another kind of terrain. Moral justifications made from here will appear to others as incomprehensible, or just plain wrong.

HABITUS

Because the subjective experience of disability is intrinsically to do with the body, the mind, and the world, and because however much its meaning is socially mediated it is also an interior phenomenon, we are left with the problem of how, practically, to get at it. How can we get a handle on whether, and in which ways, something as intangible as *what it is like to be (in) this body* modifies moral understandings? How do we begin to unravel moral understandings that are so "obvious" that people feel no need to argue for them, to others and especially not to themselves?

The analytic approach of the twentieth-century French anthropologist Pierre Bourdieu offers one way of getting some purchase on those features of life, formed at the interface between body and world, that are intrinsically hard to grasp. Bourdieu's concern is with how social understandings become part of the taken-for-granted fabric of individual lives, and how in turn the regular, everyday enactment of these understandings is absorbed by the social world. For disability theory his approach has the advantage of taking as its starting point the fully embodied subject in the social world, and of trying to avoid a dichotomization of body and environment. In contrast to much traditional philosophy of mind and cognitive science, Bourdieu says that human understanding cannot be seen solely in terms of perceptions that we receive, convert into internal representations, and ultimately articulate in words. Instead, much of our conscious reasoning emerges from a prereflexive background of meaning. Moreover, much of this background of meaning is carried by and expressed in the everyday practices of human living. These are practices that are performed by bodies, and so our bodies (their shape, how they move, the actions they perform, how they interact with material objects and with the bodies of others in various social contexts) carry elements of our understanding of ourselves and the world.

Bourdieu's concept of *habitus* refers to patterns of being and doing in the world that people acquire through becoming habituated to a particular social field. Each such field generates its own system of tacit rules governing practices and behaviors, "durable, transposable dispositions . . . [that act] as principles which generate and organize practices and representations that can be objectively adapted to their outcomes without presupposing a conscious aiming at ends" (Bourdieu 1990, 53). Habitus is pretheoretical, prereflexive knowledge that we absorb from the behavior and practices that are demonstrated, rarely articulated, by the people around us. By means of the habitus the subject acquires a set of dispositions that are manifested both physically in the bodily hexis ("a durable way of standing, speaking, walking, and thereby of thinking and feeling" [Bourdieu 1990, 69–70]), and also mentally in tendencies toward patterns of perceiving and interpreting the world. So it is not just habits of physical behavior that become deeply ingrained, but habits of thought and affect as well. Habitus then is best seen as an entanglement of physicality and mental life, and Bourdieu generally avoids talking about different aspects of the habitus separately on the grounds that to do so reinforces the view he wants to reject, that physical and mental faculties are clearly separable (Bourdieu 1993, 86). The bodily understanding of the habitus is carried not in mental representations of image or word but as a feel for the right behavior. Knowing what is fitting is what gives us the ability to function in a given social milieu without constantly and consciously thinking about it: Bourdieu described this as "the practical sense" or more evocatively as "knowing how to play the game." This kind of knowledge may never be consciously articulated (at least not in the absence of sociologists asking questions about it). Indeed, the schemes of the habitus owe their enormous potency and persistence to the fact that they operate outside the reach of conscious control.

What Bourdieu is saying is that reality is "made real," is cognitively structured, through bodily processes that originate in the social world. The sense of effortlessness—the fact that there *is* no felt sense of structuring, but rather a feeling of obvious rightness—results from being at home within a familiar habitus and indicates that the structuring of reality is not volitional. The structuring of habitus is inscribed very early on, and as a result its manifestations appear self-evident. Things out of alignment with it are obviously absurd or illogical or barbaric. This is a significantly different idea from the one that says frameworks and tacit understandings of morality *can* be clarified using intellectual skills but that people mostly lack either the skill or the will to do so (thus allowing moral philosophers to earn an honest living). Bourdieu suggests that these understandings of the right and the good are not readily accessible to conscious scrutiny from philosophers or anyone else. The habitus, prereflexive and embodied, slips under the radar of the most acute critique.

For a particular habitus to function smoothly, it must be taken for granted and people must be able to think that all its features "are in fact necessities, common sense, natural or inevitable" (Webb et al. 2002, 38–39). So habitus serves to naturalize itself and the social world that generates it. In the moral context our beliefs and values, as well as the forms of reasoning and justification that seem compelling, are cognitively structured through the habitus, but we don't (can't) see it happening.

HABITUS AND MORAL UNDERSTANDING

The understandings of the world mediated through habitus include moral understandings as well. The ethical link here is on two levels: (1) those practices that are in keeping with the habitus will be taken as both "fitting" and "morally good"; and (2) ingrained habits of feeling and thought will include moral ideas and emotions about things like the good life, responsibilities to others and how they should be fulfilled, what sorts of acts exhibit genuine moral agency, and so on. The first level takes in a mixture of social convention and ethics. It is the second sense that is most relevant to the consideration of moral choices. In one of his rare discussions of ethics Bourdieu suggests that habitus includes what he calls *ethos*, and by this he seems to mean something akin to Margaret Walker's conceptualization of everyday moral understandings: in Bourdieusian terms, a set of practices that are mobilized in situations in which ethical questions are raised (Bourdieu 1993, 86–88). Bourdieu's own words on this are worth quoting in full:

> [I]f one forgets that we may have principles in the practical state, without having a systematic morality, an ethic, one forgets that simply by asking questions, interrogating, one forces people to move from ethos to ethic; in inviting a judgment on constituted, verbalized norms, one assumes that this shift has been made. Or, in another sense, one forgets that people may prove incapable of responding to ethical problems while being quite capable of responding in practice to situations raising the corresponding questions. . . . Moreover, all the principles of choice are "embodied," turned into postures, dispositions of the body. Values are postures, gestures, ways of standing, walking, speaking. The strength of the ethos is that it is a morality made flesh. (Bourdieu 1993, 86)

The dispositions of the habitus are neither purely automatic reflexes nor propositional mental acts, but reflect some features of both. An agent's action (for example, a decision about prenatal screening) would, in a Bourdieusian frame, be a conscious decision that emerged within the dispositional constraints of habitus. The justification an agent might give for her choice and act is propositional: it can be articulated in terms of reasons. The point is that the reasons given are found compelling to the agent because of this indwelling sense of rightness and will be found convincing to others to the extent that the reasons line up with their own "durable dispositions," which cannot be articulated propositionally, or only with effort. If this is the case, it would not be surprising if anomalous embodiment generates at least some moral dispositions that fit awkwardly to the schemes of evaluation driven by the dominant habitus.

Through focusing on specific everyday practices of bodies in social contexts, Bourdieu's model offers a way of fleshing out in detail what are often frustratingly vague and general statements about the social construction of moral thinking. It enables us to ask targeted questions about how, exactly, being a person of a given gender, social class, religious milieu, or body form provides a framework around which specific moral perceptions and understandings consolidate.

HABITUS AND DISABLED MORAL UNDERSTANDING

To study the effect of embodiment in a Bourdieusian sense would be to follow how cultural rules "get into the body," progressively structuring its actions and perceptions and becoming incorporated into the manners of standing, speaking, feeling, and thinking, becoming integrated with our sense of identity. It is the dialogical embodied and social nature of the process through which habitus is generated and taken up that makes it particularly relevant to impairment's effect on the background of moral understanding. Bourdieu is trying to articulate a way in which a physical body interacts with a social world to generate meaning. The individuality of this production derives, in part, from the specifics of the body: what the constraints of biology and physics allow the body to do, and the possibilities that are open to *that* kind of body in *that* social organization. Looking at it this way means we need not agonize over whether disability is "really" a consequence of an impaired phenotype, or alternatively the result of a society's oppression. Disability becomes a way of being that arises only because of the existence of both body and world.

The question we can then ask is, what is the effect on habitus of the experience of being/having a body that is not the standard model? Bourdieu himself only really considered bodily variation in terms of gendered difference, in his examination of masculinities, or of the lives of the Kabyle women. Even this was limited, and Bourdieu has come under strong attack from feminist thinkers for this neglect. Both McCall (1992) and Lovell

(2000) argue that his work seriously downplays gender, sexuality, and ethnicity, focusing instead on social class, which he seems to consider more
foundational to the formation of habitus. It may also be that Bourdieu was
simply more comfortable dealing with class than with gender. Nevertheless,
sociologists after Bourdieu have applied his ideas to other dimensions of
social organization, so there are precedents here. To do the same thing for
the body that is impaired, however, means performing a significantly different analysis, because the processes involved are significantly different.
Small girls and boys acquire the marks of their gendered habitus very early
on, first through their immersion in their family groups and then through
repeated contacts with the wider society that schools them in gendered behaviors. One immediately obvious difference between gender and impairment, then, is that with a few exceptions—a dwarf growing up in a family
where other members have restricted growth, or a hearing-impaired child in
a Deaf family and surrounded by the Deaf world—most children with a
physical impairment will grow up in settings where their particular body is
not normative. In fact, it is likely to be the case that the majority of people
with impairments do not have a rightful habitus, other than what might
best be described as the habitus of failure. This would be, in Bourdieu's
terms, an ill-fitting set of dispositions that are generated by being chroni-
cally unable to keep the tacit rules of normal comportment, timing, speech,
and so on. The physical environment, everyday objects that need to be manipulated, how people move around, how they communicate with each
other—in cases of impairment, few of these will accommodate the specific
features of the child's functioning. Hence to a greater or lesser extent there
will be persistent mismatch between the demands of the prevailing habitus
and what a person's body is in practice able to do.
    When Jacqueline Rose writes that "most women do not painlessly slip
into their roles as women" (1983, 9), she means that in every society there
is a gendered habitus available to women, but that because of its oppressive nature—because it reflects the expectations of a dominant group that
is gendered differently—it is not taken on/generated without a struggle. In
an interview with Terry Eagleton, Bourdieu said, "The doxic attitude does
not mean happiness: it means bodily submission, unconscious submission, which may indicate a lot of internalized tension, a lot of bodily suffering. . . . [T]his smooth working of habitus . . . helps people to adjust, but
it causes internalized contradictions" (Bourdieu and Eagleton 1992, 121).
These struggles are the pain that Rose points to. Nevertheless, and despite
those contradictions, there does exist a recognized way of being a woman
in the world, and even of being a morally "good" woman. The struggle and
contradiction for disabled people are somewhat different. Like women,
members of the working class, or black people, they don't do any painless
slipping, but in their case for the reason that although the dominant soci-

ety is likely to have social spaces for disabled people, its repertoire does not
include habitus in which the disabled person can "effortlessly" play the
same game as people with normative embodiments. Bourdieu puts it like
this: "The degree to which one can abandon oneself to the automatisms of
practical sense obviously varies with the situation and area of activity, but
also with the position occupied in social space: it is likely that those who
are in 'their right place' in the social world can abandon or entrust themselves . . . to their dispositions" (Bourdieu 2000, 163). This does not mean
that disabled people are unable to play the majority game at all: they
patently can, and in fact this is fundamentally what is going on when disabled people engage with others in ways that enable those others to say,
But I never think of you as disabled. What they often cannot do is play it with
the same degree of unthinking ease. The condition of not sharing the
effortless habitus of normal embodiment is central to what disability is all
about.

Note that this does not mean that women effortlessly share the *dominant*
habitus either. I am suggesting rather that widespread recognition of a social
role, even a marginalized one, leads to the stabilization of the habitus that
goes with it. It may be constrained and inferior to another (a male habitus,
for example, or an upper-class one) but it does at least exist, and it is possible to acquire it, and in doing so to have a home in the world. This is not the
case for impairment in most contexts of contemporary Western society.

For Bourdieu, an important aspect of generating habitus is its inscription
on the body: "Our habitus is at once produced and expressed through our
movements, gestures, facial expressions, manners, ways of walking, and
ways of looking at the world" (Moi 1991, 1031). What follows from this is
the profound significance of having a body that fails to follow those rules.
The training that inculcates an unspoken understanding of legitimate ways
to (re)present the body to ourselves and others also produces an equally
unspoken, but equally powerful, repertoire of *illegitimate* modes of bodily
representation. Indeed, we might want to ask whether one reason that bodily difference disturbs people so much is that it reminds them, at some
level, of the contingency of the dispositions of the habitus that they are normally able to take as self-evident. In the early 1960s, an estimated ten thou-
sand babies worldwide were born with limb anomalies as a result of their
mothers' being prescribed the drug thalidomide during pregnancy (thalidomide turned out to be a potent teratogen). When these infants began to
walk and reach for objects, they were usually provided with prosthetic
limbs. This was done in the face of accumulating evidence that the children
could often devise their own way of moving about or manipulating objects
using the limbs they had in unusual but serviceable ways. They frequently
found prostheses awkward, sometimes spectacularly so. Alison Lapper[6] describes how "the intention was to enable us to do the normal things that

people in the outside world did, but they also wanted to help us look as normal as possible. . . . It was all very admirable but the final results, the awkward arm-substitutes, were ridiculous . . . because it was virtually impossible to use them for the purpose for which they were intended. . . . If a stranger had walked into our dining room during a typical mealtime they . . . would have seen some of us chasing the same bit of food round and round a plate without ever getting hold of it. I never managed to eat any of my meals hot for that reason. Others would have succeeded in grabbing a piece of something but then would whack themselves in the chin or eye when they tried to lift it up to their mouth. Yet others would accidentally flip their food down the table or across it into someone's lap or face. . . . By the time I was seven or eight the authorities had accepted that the experiment wasn't working and they more or less gave up asking us to use artificial arms. Instead a knife and spoon were strapped directly to my stumps" (Lapper 2005, 33–36).

The resistance to these children developing their own way of being in the world was enormously strong. And it remains so: as I was revising this chapter in summer 2007, a woman in the United States was suing McDonald's for damages because of the behavior of its employees at one branch. As a result of the genetic condition Holt-Oram syndrome, Dawn Larson has no upper limbs. She steered her car into a drive-in McDonald's with her feet and used a foot to pick up her order. The less-than-sensitive reaction of the counter staff—"Girl, what's the matter with you? You ain't got no arms! Let me see your arms"—(Pallasch 2007) underlines just how uncomfortable it makes people feel to see others using the "wrong" limbs, or walking on their bottom and not on legs. The discomfort and the resistance almost certainly derive a great deal of their power from the operations of the prevailing habitus and its internalized rules. The unexamined, taken for grantedness of background understandings can be unsettled when either the objective social conditions change, or when subjective expectations are, for whatever reason, challenged (being confronted with a customer picking up a bag with her foot, for example). It is in such moments of conflict that critical reflection on doxic assumptions becomes possible.

HABITUS AND THE DEAF WORLD

It may be true that if we "conceive of the Deaf as being members of a linguistic and cultural minority, our moral landscape should be altered" (Crouch 1997, 17). The cast list of our mental moral theater would then include actors who were culturally Deaf as well as actors who were disabled by hearing impairment. Still, if a person's moral understanding is generated from cumulative social, embodied experiences, a rational reconceptualization of hearing impairment would not mean we ended up owning the *same* understanding as culturally Deaf people. In the previous chapter I argued that an outsider's ability to project herself imaginatively into the moral world of another person is more limited than we think, especially when important aspects of her embodied experience are different. Here I want to see whether a consideration of habitus might be one route to grasping why many (though certainly not all) people in the Deaf world find a preference for having a hearing-impaired child to be natural and intuitively obvious, even if they themselves would not choose to act on it. I will draw from ethnographic, sociological, and autobiographical accounts of the Deaf experience to demonstrate that such experience may contribute to a "Deaf habitus" in which certain practices and values are ranked differently than in the dominant hearing world.

For culturally Deaf people—who, it must be remembered, are a minority of hearing-impaired people[7]—the Deaf social world generates a particular habitus shaped not just by bodily constraint (ears that do not work like audionormals') but also by the sociocultural traditions of the community. Many of the distinctive features of this world are to do with the parameters of communicating in Sign. Most native Signers, for example, have a characteristic, and to the hearing world unusual or even grotesque, animation of face and body movements. Compared to speech, Sign is an *embodied*, physically expressive mode of communication. As Oliver Sacks notes, "Signing . . . is a voice given a special force because it utters itself, so immediately, with the body. One can have or imagine disembodied speech, but one cannot have disembodied Sign" (Sacks 1989, 199). Like any spoken language, Sign also has a set of subtle rules that enable its users to play the game. There are rules about using the direction of the gaze or the space around the body, and others that are not primarily about gestures or grammatical structure, but such things as the signals that manage turn-taking in conversation, for example. Like their equivalents in spoken language, rules like these are not normally handed on explicitly in codified form, except where an adult is learning Sign as a foreign language. Mostly, they are incorporated by repeated performance, the "structured structures functioning as structuring structures" of Bourdieu's opaque terminology.

But although Sign is important, a point that is frequently missed by both deaf and hearing commentators is that being culturally Deaf means more than simply using gestural instead of spoken language. Not all the dispositions of a Deaf habitus may be traced back to the demands of signing. Other characteristics reflect the *prediscursive* features of a world in which most stimuli are visual or tactile rather than auditory. In a Deaf context, for example, people tend to use physical contact to a degree that is unusual in the hearing world. To attract each other's attention or let someone know that a person has entered the room, touching or gentle tapping (among children and adolescents it may not always be so gentle) are generally quite acceptable (Metzger and Bahan 2001). This can create difficulties for a culturally Deaf person in the hearing world, which has different rules about acceptable touch and proximity. Physical space and contact are immensely sensitive areas of nonverbal communication, and getting the rules wrong can be perceived as rude or even threatening.

That we can legitimately speak of a Deaf habitus is indicated by the way some Deaf people describe their experience in the ethnographic and autobiographical literature. Deaf memoirs are full of metaphors of being at home that suggest a state of understanding and of being understood without needing to think twice about it: a space, unlike the hearing world, where Deaf people know and can follow the implicit rules of the game. In his pioneer sociology of deafness, Higgins concludes that "within deaf communities . . . a sense of belonging and wholeness is achieved which is not found [by deaf people] among the hearing" (Higgins 1980, 76). He reports his informants' saying things like "most of my friends are deaf, I feel more comfortable with them. Well, we have the same feelings. We are more comfortable with each other" (42), or "when I saw these people (at a deaf organization) I knew I belonged to their world. I didn't belong in the hearing world" (38).

The Deaf habitus can be a profound mismatch to the hearing world. Practices that are unnoticed because they do not stand out in the Deaf world become stigmatizing elsewhere, and part of the discomfort for culturally Deaf people in the hearing world is that rigorous self-monitoring is necessary in order to "pass." Lou Ann Walker describes how this self-control over behaviors that were ingrained and automatic altered the comportment of her Deaf family: "[Outside the Deaf world], whoever it was doing the talking had a power over us. Our signs were small and timid, and our faces were almost immobile. But when we were at home alone, the five of us were transformed and the signing was large and generous" (Walker 1986, 108).

Unlike the hearing world, the Deaf world provides Deaf people with a habitus in which they feel at home and where the obvious does not have to be explained. Paul Preston's interviews with Deaf and mixed families include one with Sandra, a young deaf woman who puts it like this: "Usually I understand why a deaf person did so and so. I can understand why they did it. But I can't explain to hearing people. Like, when I saw it, it didn't look wrong to me. I understood just fine, but to hearing people it looks real strange. I don't even think about it, don't think anything about it. That's just how deaf people are, no big deal. And then they [hearing people] look at me like (sign "gape" and "dumb"). They want an answer. But I don't have a black and white answer for them" (Preston 2001, 14). It is characteristic of the operation of habitus that not only are things obvious, they are so obvious, for so long, that we lack the language to explain them.

Habitus is a function of both the body that experiences and the socio-cultural world in which experience happens, and so to explore its moral ramifications fully requires detailed examination of the worlds that produce the particularities of experience. As I said, debate about Duchesneau-McCullough and related cases is marked by the neglect of the social world in which those moral understandings were shaped and decisions made. I want to sketch out some features of the culturally Deaf world that seem pertinent to evaluating these stories.

Deaf culture—if we accept that there is such a thing—is distinctive in that, unlike other linguistic and ethnic cultures to which it is compared by both Deaf and hearing commentators, it is maintained and transmitted predominantly horizontally through peer contacts, and not vertically down through the family. As hearing impairment is generally not genetic, most hearing-impaired children (the figure commonly given is 90 percent) have hearing parents, while in most cases two deaf adults will have hearing children together unless the parental deafness is due to the same genetic lesion. The transmission of audiological deafness *and* of Deaf culture, then, is usually disrupted in each generation. In the past this led to the sociological novelty that the chief conduits for Deaf identity were institutional, mainly schools for the deaf or Deaf clubs (Jennifer Harris 1995, 121–40), and in fact until quite recently older deaf people would still give the name of their school when asked where they "came from": the school for the deaf was their point of entry into their self-identification as Deaf (Padden and Humphries 2005).[8] More than one author has suggested that the Deaf world has a stronger sense of its group identity than the hearing world (Jennifer Harris 1995; Preston 2001). This strength of group identification is a common feature of socially marginalized groups. The majority culture is unlikely to distinguish the equivalent feature as an identifier, because for most hearing people, there is no such thing as "the hearing world." There is just *the world*; because being hearing is the norm, it is not recognized as a marker for group identity.

Group identification is probably enhanced by the fact that even today, for many hearing-impaired children and adolescents the Deaf world is a *found* community. Many Deaf memoirs are structured around a narrative of "coming home" after years of isolation and frustration because of the impossibility of hearing speech. The strength of Deaf identification is illustrated by occasional references in the literature to instances where Deaf identity overrides other identifications, such as religion: Higgins, for instance, reports members of a synagogue for the deaf preferring to donate items to a bazaar supporting a Lutheran deaf church than to another synagogue for hearing Jews (Higgins 1980, 39). Some years ago I undertook a study, together with colleagues in Switzerland, of how relevant ethical issues in gene therapy are perceived by different involved agents (Scully et al. 2004). During the study we interviewed people with a range of chronic illnesses and disabilities, including some hearing-impaired people recruited from a local Deaf social club. These participants strongly identified with the Deaf world—so strongly in fact that some of them, when asked to state their nationality, gave "the Deaf world" in place of "Switzerland." And almost without exception, those we interviewed opposed the future use of somatic gene therapies to treat hearing impairment in an adult. The reason they gave was that it would sever a person's existing connections with the Deaf world, and they saw this as a central ethical concern.

Deaf culture is transmitted vertically, through the family, only in the small proportion of cases where both parents have the same genetic basis for their hearing impairment. The rarity of this makes deaf children of deaf parents, the so-called deaf of deaf, peculiarly significant within the Deaf world. In the past they have provided a crucial element of cultural continuity within their home environment and thereby the means to pass cultural knowledge on to deaf children from hearing families (Preston 2001, 71). Within the Deaf world, then, the deaf of deaf may be considered a kind of elite. An article on Deaf activism in the United States quoted one such woman as saying, "I've always said that I'd get to the top and open as many doors as I could for the whole Deaf community," while another remarked on his extended lineage with considerable pride: "My father and my grandfather went to Lexington [a school for the deaf in the United States]. I am Deaf of Deaf of Deaf" (Solomon 1994).

A person's social context is formed not just by the network of relationships in which she is immersed, but also by the way those relationships are socially organized according to status and hierarchies of various kinds. So for people whose primary social context is the Deaf world, it will be far from intuitively obvious that being hearing impaired within a hearing-impaired family and Deaf social network is worse than being hearing within a hearing-impaired family. Furthermore, from a Deaf perspective it will not be obvious that such a child would suffer more social disadvantages than a hearing child. Recall that most commentators on the Duchesneau-McCullough case, working from the standpoint of a hearing or, in some cases, deafened person, assumed that hearing impairment entailed a substantial reduction in the sum of abilities, and also in social competence and status. They focused on the limitations faced by the deaf child that a hearing child would not encounter: as Davis put it, the damage done to the child's right to an open future. Revealingly, without exception commentators failed to raise the possibility that a hearing child might also face barriers growing up in a deaf familial and social context. Yet there is sociological and anecdotal evidence to suggest that the life of a hearing child within a deaf family is not automatically unproblematic (Bull 1998; Singleton and Tittle 2000; Preston 2001). Among the issues that have been identified are the child's awareness and negotiation of family difference; use in an age-inappropriate way as an interpreter and "cultural mediator" (Preston 2001, 96–103; Couser 1997, 250); difficulties in developing an individual identity when that is overwhelmed by the perceived categorical difference between hearing and Deaf members of the family;[9] mixed loyalties between Deaf and hearing worlds, and difficulty belonging to both; or experience of deferred stigmatization. Now clearly these problems are not inevitable, and they may not be experienced as problems, or not overwhelming ones anyway, by the people concerned. The point is rather that issues like these, which are key data in weighing up exactly what kind of harm or good we are talking about, were not discussed, while the potential difficulties faced by a deaf child in a hearing world were repeatedly rehearsed. A certain form of embodiment is not only taken to be normative, but to be universally unproblematic, irrespective of context. That a normal embodiment is still a body, with embodied limitations, essentially fades from sight as relevant to ethical judgment; it's as if there is no embodiment there at all, or none worth taking note of.

A final relevant element is the Deaf community's awareness of its history. Today many hearing-impaired people have a historical narrative[10] that highlights the pioneer deaf educators[11] of the seventeenth to nineteenth centuries, a period in which Deaf schools were founded and public and philosophical interest in signed languages grew, followed by the turning point of the Milan Congress of educators of the deaf in 1880, after which education aimed at integration into the hearing world came to dominate. For something like the next hundred years, schools for the deaf operated with a strong, often exclusive focus on oralism and the suppression of sign language. Although this was undoubtedly beneficial to many hearing-impaired children, for others it meant being cut off from a supportive signing community. Scholars of Deaf history have also traced the efforts of twentieth-century eugenic movements in Europe and North America to discourage hearing-impaired people from having children, efforts that ultimately led to German National Socialism's active euthanasia program and the attempted elimination of the genetically defective, including hearing-impaired people (Kerr and Shakespeare 2002; Ryan and Schuchman 2002).

Against this sociocultural and historical background, then, Deaf people define deviance from a different center (Couser 1997, 224). To those who think of themselves as a cultural or linguistic minority—and not all culturally Deaf people would agree with this description either—it makes no sense to claim that "choosing" deafness violates the child's future autonomy. Choosing deafness, they might say, is rather like choosing to practice your Judaism, or to send your child to a Rudolf Steiner school: a cultural choice that closes down some options, for sure, but opens up others that are equally or perhaps more valuable. Aware that by objective criteria many deaf people perform poorly in terms of education or employment, they may ascribe this to the negative effects of discrimination (inappropriate schooling, lack of sign language interpreters in higher education and the workplace) rather than the impairment itself. Some Deaf people might then choose to avoid deafness in their children, to protect them from these disadvantages, rather as parents might elect not to practice a minority religion so that their children can fit better into the mainstream culture. But others would believe that difficulties caused by societal prejudice do not constitute *good enough* grounds for preferring a hearing over a hearing-impaired child.

CARING FOR THE CHILD/CARING FOR THE COMMUNITY

Some commentators criticized Duchesneau and McCullough, and by implication any disabled parents who express a preference for offspring with "their" impairment, for egotistically wanting "a child like themselves." This is a complex point. For starters, it's worth bearing in mind that, broadly speaking, we think this is a legitimate desire for any parent to have. We assume, for example, that parents would rather have their own genetically related offspring than adopt someone else's; we find the preference for genetic relationship a natural one. Yet a genetic relationship per se is invisible. It has to be experienced phenotypically, so what we really mean by "genetically related to" is "looks and behaves like" its parents.

Wanting a child "like myself" can be straight narcissism, but it can also be lots more. It can reflect the parents' concern about being able to foster emotional bonds, for example. Parents may believe that they can best care for a child who is more like themselves: that they will be better able to empathize, anticipate its needs, and provide appropriate guidance as it grows, than for a hearing child whose experiences and position in the world are too different from their own (Scully 2006b). Paul Preston quotes a deaf mother describing the birth of her hearing daughter: "When Barbara was born, it wasn't until about three days later that I had this funny feeling about her. . . . [When I discovered she was hearing] I couldn't believe it! I was really upset. I thought, Oh my God . . . what on earth am I going to do with her? I don't even know how to talk to her. . . . *I wanted to be close to my children . . . I worried that we would never connect, or that we would drift apart*" (Preston 2001, 17; my italics).

Deaf parents might also feel that a child who fits into the surrounding community will benefit from having an easier time growing up. The same might be said of a black child growing up in a predominantly white area. This cuts both ways, of course, because hearing-impaired children will inevitably live in a larger hearing society that extends beyond the Deaf community and in which, ideally, they will have a place as adults. Still, there are families—like those of Duchesneau and McCullough—in which numerous family members, and the community within which the family socializes, are all hearing impaired; here the parents might believe that a child does best as a full member of such a community, and so will be better prepared, psychologically and socially, for his or her encounter with the wider world. An analogy here might be expat Britons living in Zurich who work and socialize almost exclusively with other expats and who therefore choose to send their children to the local English-speaking or international school, arguing that it will better equip them with the confidence and competencies to manage in either Britain or Switzerland.

Whether or not it is true that dissimilarity disrupts the proper formation of the parent-child bond (and we can all summon enough personal examples of wildly dysfunctional "natural" families, and flourishing families of the very unlike, to reserve judgment on that), or that children will develop more confidently in a community where they don't stand out as anomalous, the point is that the form this concern takes is more other-directed than the base egotistical desire to create something in one's own impaired image. It is interesting that Robert Crouch picks up the analogous reasoning used by hearing parents wondering if their hearing-impaired child would benefit from a prelingual cochlear implant: "Struck by the otherness of the life that they imagine their child will lead . . . parents will usually choose [an implant] . . . to prevent a chasm from opening up between them and their child (so that their child is in the same community as they are)" (Crouch 1997, 15). The desire for parents and child to share a culture is seen as justified in this case, while it is condemned as selfish or egotistical when used by Deaf parents. The condemnation is not of the desire itself, but of the wish for physical or behavioral or cultural similarity to outweigh the welfare of the child. Yet as we have seen, that weighing-up may just not work from a culturally Deaf perspective.

By prioritizing the relational context (Rehmann-Sutter 1999), it becomes possible to trace how these parental choices are rooted in care: both the physical and emotional care for the child, and caring for its future in ensuring it will grow up as a valued member of a flourishing community rather than what they might fear as being on its periphery, or lost between Deaf and hearing worlds. This would mean that, in having a preference for a hearing-impaired child and, within limits that are still contested, acting on that preference, Deaf parents might not only claim to be showing an attitude of care toward their own child, but also toward not-yet-existing hearing-impaired people. The genetic choice to have hearing-impaired children has been described as sacrificing those children's open futures for the sake of a putative Deaf community. There are large debates here about whether cultures or communities are valuable in themselves, or only for what they give their members. Although the loss of Deaf culture might be a sadness if we consider cultures as good in themselves, Neil Levy argues that if cultures are instrumentally not intrinsically valuable, "there ought to be no ethical problems in allowing [Deaf culture] to die, so long as its members are at least as well off in terms of the goods which cultures make available to their members as they would otherwise have been" (Levy 2002b, 136). But because the Deaf culture is not equivalent to other linguistic or ethnic minorities, there are harder consequences of its loss. If the Cornish or Rumantsch languages or cultures die out, the children growing up in those areas in the future will still flourish, adapting to the prevailing language and culture (probably English and German respectively). This won't work for future hearing-impaired people—not just children born deaf, but deafened adolescents and adults—many of whom, even supported by lipreading and other aids to hearing, including cochlear implants, will still be less than fully competent in a solely hearing world.

So the preference for hearing-impaired children can be redescribed as showing responsibility toward future hearing-impaired children and adults, who will inevitably come into existence,[12] to ensure the survival of a socially flourishing and politically strong Deaf community of which they can be part. Different moral understandings drive those two different descriptions, and their evaluation pivots on how one pictures the ethical relationship between individual and community in general, and how this one particular community is valued.

Two things need to be underlined before we move on. One is that in my discussion of the Deaf community I have focused on a minority of a minority and simplified the real complexity of the relationships between different kinds of hearing-impaired people. As Mairian Corker and others have demonstrated, considerable oversimplification is involved when "Deaf" and "deaf," or "Deaf" and "hearing," are placed in simple opposition. These categorizations either leave out (or force uncomfortably in) the signing deaf who nevertheless do not consider themselves part of a "Deaf community," moderately hearing-impaired people who can sign and also function well in hearing contexts, or nonsigning audiologically deaf people who can use hearing aids or cochlear implants to participate fully in "phonocentric" or hearing society (Corker 2002). Relationships between these and the "Deaf" or "hearing" can be theoretically contested, but in the real lives of hearing-impaired people they are, on the whole, managed without too much difficulty. They are dynamic relationships too, as new kinds of involvements are facilitated through technological and social change (Chorost 2005). An example of the former would be the rise of real-time communication through nonaural means (texting, e-mail, instant messaging), and of the latter the interest of hearing people in the nonhearing world *as* a distinct culture (and the associated issues of exoticization and romanticization, which I have no space to go into here). Second, none of what I have said here should be taken as a *plaidoyer* for the genetic selection of impairment. It should be clear that I do not think that knowing more about the bases of moral understandings will give answers, or easier answers, to ethical questions. I do think that it will help give better answers, though, and one way in which it does this is by starting to denaturalize standard frameworks of judgment. By this I mean that focusing on the Deaf, or disabled, habitus looks at only half the problem. I have concentrated on the Deaf habitus as constituting a particular set of moral dispositions that are manifest, among other things, in the choices that some members of the Deaf community make. Inevitably, though, the same holds for the hearing world. The habitus of the hearing world (the dispositions and so on carried by its members) is, like all habitus, a function both of the social world and the bodies active in it; and, again like all habitus, it serves to naturalize the background assumptions of the hearing world. And so the assumptions fade from sight as things that might need justification: they *just are so.* What also escapes notice is that descriptive and evaluative strategies are cut to fit comfortably with the demands of the hearing world. As Bourdieu puts it, "When people only have to let their habitus follow its natural bent in order to comply with the immanent necessity of the field and satisfy the demands contained within it . . . they are not at all aware of fulfilling a duty, still less of seeking to maximize their (specific) profit. So they enjoy the additional profit of seeing themselves and being seen as totally disinterested" (Bourdieu 1993, 76).

EMBODIED THINKING

Is it at all imaginable that being habituated to the Deaf rather than the hearing world means socioculturally Deaf people *think* differently, in some respects, from people who hear? At first sight the idea may not seem very likely, and even offensive, if we make the mistake of assuming that "differently" means "less well." Disability activism has worked hard over the last fifty or so years to ensure that disabled people's moral and political equality with nondisabled people is recognized. Disabled people would rightly reject anything that calls that equality into question. So I will reiterate here, as I do throughout the book, that highlighting difference neither implies nor justifies inequality.

The neurologist Oliver Sacks has suggested, although with no empirical or experimental basis that I know of, that because it is through inner speech—that is, silent talking to oneself—that a child develops a sense of her own subjectivity, the differences between speech and Sign may give rise to "a unique and untranslatable, hypervisual cognitive style" that could contribute to a distinct "Deaf subjectivity" (Sacks 1989, 73, 74-75n). On the basis of the available evidence (or lack of it) we might be reluctant to go quite that far. Still, there are some indications that at least parts of the Deaf world feel that "Deaf ways" and "hearing ways" of thinking are sometimes not the same. In American Sign Language (ASL), a hearing-impaired person who acts out the values of the hearing world is indicated by a sign that is glossed as THINK-HEARING, meaning that she "thinks like a hearing person" (Kannapell 1982, 24), and this is usually meant as an insult (Padden and Humphries 1994, 52). And Higgins quotes a deaf signing woman who has difficulties discussing things with oral deaf people, not because the people themselves are difficult, but because, she says, "Their arguments seem strange" (Higgins 1980, 66).

What the Bourdieusian framework of habitus and field offers is a way of analyzing an individual's interpretative framework within her embodied and social context, avoiding or minimizing the dichotomy of body and world, and offering a degree of distance to help compare different interpretative frameworks, to analyze their development and the power relations and strategies that enable one or some to override others. Bourdieu, however, has been criticized on a lot of fronts, and one of the most cogent criticisms is that the heuristic of the habitus does not provide a mechanism for what it says takes place. Although trying to work through the dialectical relationship of body and world, Bourdieu nevertheless remains an anthropologist with an anthropologist's interest in external practices, skipping blithely over the mechanics of how bodily social experience might be internalized into mental processes. In the next chapter I move on to ask what sorts of perceptual, cognitive, or affective steps might be involved in this internalization, and what sort of difference bodily anomaly might make.

NOTES

1. It is arguable that the amount of bioethical debate of this and analogous cases is completely disproportionate. The number of cases involved remains small. In a survey of the practices of IVF clinics in the United States, Baruch et al. (2008) mention (without giving further details) that 3 percent of IVF-PGD clinics reported having provided PGD to couples to select for a disability.

2. That is, in the reputable academic and media debate. The wilder fringes of discussion, available online, were much readier to argue either that the two women should not have reproduced on eugenic grounds because they were genetically deaf and therefore defective, or that the fact that it was two *women* demonstrated the homosexual agenda to exploit reproductive technologies to take over the world. I'm paraphrasing here.

3. Remember that Duchesneau and McCullough were only increasing the chances of having a hearing-impaired child, not determining it with certainty. Other techniques, such as PGD, incorporating a test for a well-characterized locus associated with genetic deafness would have been much more reliable.

4. Though one has to ask how much, put like this, it differs from the way that cumulative educational and social policy choices have the same effect.

5. Clearly, these arguments are applicable beyond prenatal genetic testing or donor insemination. They have also cropped up in the debate over giving cochlear implants to prelingually deaf children. In theory, cochlear implants have the potential to offer (a form of) hearing to profoundly deaf children who are unable to benefit from conventional hearing aids, an intervention that, it is recognized, "can *determine* community membership" (Crouch 1997) (and by implication the futures open to the child).

6. Note, however, that Lapper's phocomelia, although similar in effect, was of unknown aetiology and not the result of thalidomide.

7. The Royal National Institute for the Deaf estimates that of the 8,945,000 deaf and hard-of-hearing people in the United Kingdom there are approximately 50,000 users of British Sign Language who would consider themselves part of the culturally Deaf world.

8. The significance of the Deaf school to the perpetuation of the community lies behind the resistance of many Deaf activists to mainstreaming in education, that is, the policy of prioritizing the integration of children with impairments into standard schools. From the Deaf point of view the result is further dilution and fragmentation of the sites of Deaf culture.

9. "Paradoxically, within a community of shared identity, individual differences can emerge—identities that are not restricted to a single, all-encompassing feature" (Preston 2001, 89).

10. I leave aside here the question of how historically accurate or oversimplified this narrative really is.

11. Accounts of their work can be found in Rée (1999) and Lane (1992).

12. Even if in some future world all forms of genetic hearing impairment were identified, and familial transmission prevented, there would remain nonfamilial genetic mutations to give rise "unexpectedly" to deaf children, plus children whose hearing function is damaged through neonatal or childhood illness or accident.

5

Thinking through the Variant Body

"Marginality" thus means something altogether different to me from what it means to social theorists. It is no metaphor for the power relations between one group of human beings and another, but a literal description of where I stand (figuratively speaking): over here, on the edge, out of bounds, beneath your notice. I embody the metaphors.

—Nancy Mairs

Bourdieu's theory of habitus provides one approach to conceptualizing the contribution of the body to moral understanding. It is a fruitful approach, up to a point. But if we want to examine in finer detail the difference having/being a phenotypically variant body makes, habitus and the associated concepts of social field and hexis start to look less helpful. Bourdieu fails to take his account of body/world beyond the social interaction of subjects, the habits and practices that enable them to thrive in social groups. He theorizes that bodily encounters with others are taken up into a subject's dispositions of thought; he says nothing about the neurophysiological *mechanisms* that would make this happen. As an anthropologist (although claimed by sociologists for their own), Bourdieu is just not bothered about the cogs and wheels.

The philosopher Maurice Merleau-Ponty's work, by contrast, addresses directly the most primordial interactions between the body and its physical surroundings. Although Merleau-Ponty's approach prioritizes the individual perspective in these interactions, it can be placed alongside the more socially mediated structuring of thought that interested Bourdieu. Anthropologist Bourdieu and philosopher Merleau-Ponty share an abiding concern with the ontological and epistemological relationships between the self, the mind, the body, and the surrounding world with its objects and subjects. Both struggle to trace these relationships without falling back into the traditional analytic dichotomies of mind/body, subject/object, or interior/exterior. For both of them the self is not mind *or* body, subject *or* object, but it is also more than a vague area of overlap between the two. Being a self in the world is a realm of experience generated dynamically by the inescapable intertwining of both terms. What differentiates Bourdieu and Merleau-Ponty are their chief domains of interest, which in turn marshal their theoretical standpoints and the directions in which they look for their data.

In this chapter I want first to examine Merleau-Ponty's phenomenological approach to the thinking body for what it offers the analysis of phenotypic variation in moral understanding. I will be arguing for its usefulness, even though (as feminist critics have shown for gender) Merleau-Ponty's work pays less attention to embodied difference as a topic in itself. In part because of the limited neurological knowledge of his time, however, Merleau-Ponty ultimately does not provide a completely satisfying theory of the epistemic consequences of bodily variation, and at this point I turn to recent work in neuroscience that intriguingly substantiates and extends some of Merleau-Ponty's philosophical claims. Research into what is called *embodied cognition* provides some support for the point that both Bourdieu and Merleau-Ponty, in their different ways, try to make, and that the Western epistemological tradition finds unfamiliar: that the organic reality of the body and its processes is important to abstract thinking, including thinking about ethics.

THE THINKING BODY

In chapter 1 I suggested that a phenomenological intelligence about disability, understanding the experience of disability from the inside, is essential to inform ethical judgments about impairment. The phenomenological style of doing philosophy tries to give an account of reality through the way that objects, persons, or events appear to the consciousness of the experiencer. It is not concerned, as other branches of philosophy are, with providing a coherent, abstract metastructuring of that reality. Although Merleau-Ponty is usually classed as a phenomenologist, his methodological approach differs radically from his phenomenological predecessors and contemporaries. Brentano, Husserl, and Heidegger struggled to get at the truth of being-in-the-world through the knowledge of phenomena, but paid little attention to concretizing the body as the medium through which phenomena become known. Inevitably, then, they downplayed the way that being-in-the-world is noded in the body, with all the starkly biological particularities that entails.[1] By contrast, Merleau-Ponty starts from the position that the embodied processes of perception and motility are central to the phenomenological grasp of being-in-the-world. He was therefore open to moves in the physiological psychology of his day, which is one reason why his thinking can still dialogue with today's science of cognition.

A sense of the irreducible intercalation of mind, body, and world, counter to centuries of dualistic thinking, is gaining ground within the disciplines that address questions of consciousness and cognition. What we call *experience* is an uptake of the reality that emerges in the interplay of body and environment. That we as subjects are in a position to notice events at all, and that those events have meaning to us, are the consequence of capacities of mind, but capacities that are dependent on functions (like perception) mediated by the physical body. Traditional cognitive science and philosophy favor the kind of epistemology Charles Taylor has called "mediational,"[2] an epistemology in which our knowledge of reality is achieved through the construction of distinct interior mental representations of what's going on "out there." It involves the separation of immaterial mind and material body, and a further split between the interior representations of the mind and the "real" world outside. A lot of twentieth-century psychology, philosophy of mind, and cognitive science has rested on a picture in which the body lumbers about the world receiving sensory stimuli, leaving the mind to make sense of it all through some translational process and do its best to control the body's acts. In this picture, the body *itself* is not of major interest, except as a kind of machine for generating and housing representations of external phenomena.

So when Merleau-Ponty and the phenomenologists who follow him suggest that the human body is the *basis* of the mind, it is a bit of a departure from tradition. By saying that the mind is embodied, Merleau-Ponty means that mental life is a function of the kinetic and sensory relations between the fleshly body and its setting. Thinking of all kinds emerges as a product of these relations. This product is initially prelinguistic and precognitive, the "primary consciousness" apparent in our ability to get around in the world without actively thinking about it all the time (for instance, walking along without consciously registering the obstacles to be avoided). What Merleau-Ponty means by "mind" is primarily this prereflective knowing, prior to the development of conscious rational thought and representation. Nevertheless, he also holds that the body is the basis for other forms of higher-order thinking, including abstract thought and imagination, which he places firmly secondary to embodied preconscious processes. Thought is not a set of propositions structured by a mind distinct from the body. On the contrary, it is bodily actions or habits that make thinking possible in the first place. And so the body and its habitual actions constitute forms of knowledge about how to be: how to be human beings, and how to be particular kinds of human beings in particular social settings.

Getting a Grip on Things

Merleau-Ponty's special contribution to phenomenological theorizing of the impaired body is to offer a description of the interdependence of *primary* experiences of embodied human life—sensation, perception, and motion, an interdependence that points to how they might go on to ground thought. Perception is not straightforwardly about the body receiving information about the world, but is also how the body inhabits it. In *The Phenomenology of Perception*, Merleau-Ponty was at pains to define vision, for example, not as stimuli falling on a receptive apparatus, but as a complex set of active relationships. Perception is not just a matter of sensory organs being passively activated, but neither is it a mental process of decoding sensory information. The collaboration between perceptual and motor processes is best seen, Merleau-Ponty suggests, as one way in which the body has an intentional (object-directed) grip on its physical and social environment:

> My body is geared onto the world [some translations have "has a grip on the world"] when my perception presents me with a spectacle as varied and as clearly articulated as possible, and when my motor intentions, as they unfold, receive the responses they expect from the world. This maximum sharpness of perception and action points clearly to a perceptual *ground*, a basis of my life, a general setting in which my body can coexist with the world. (Merleau-Ponty 2002, 292)

For embodied entities, being-in-the-world means constantly striving (although mostly unaware of doing so) to achieve the best possible grip on it. And Merleau-Ponty locates this process exactly and concretely in the mechanics of sensory input and motor responses. The perceptual milieu necessarily instructs bodily orientation, movements, and skills. Through our engagement in the range of everyday activities, from the simplest to the most complex, we learn that there are bodily attitudes that give us a "best grip" on things. For example, most of us learn the stance that keeps us upright and poised within the gravitational field. We discover by trial and error that there are comportments that help us listen or observe or concentrate. Perception and action are therefore essential collaborators with each other from our earliest embodied moments. The idea that perception and movement are constitutive of each other, not two distinct functions, dissolves the traditional conceptual split between the mental and the material.

Prelinguistic, Nonconceptual Content

This phenomenology of origins digs away at the world of perceptions and understandings that exist before words and interpretations become possible, or even necessary. Merleau-Ponty's achievement was to see the need to struggle, even with qualified success, to articulate forms of experience that are by definition hard if not impossible to bring to speech: what is going on for the body, prior to any form of words. Most philosophy, and most moral philosophy, and hence ethical analysis, deals in rational thought processes, and the tools of these trades are words and concepts. But rational discourse is often inappropriate for what Merleau-Ponty calls the *pre-predicative life of consciousness*, the primordial layer of experiences that are normally never put into propositional subject/predicate form.

What is distinctive about Merleau-Ponty's claim is his insistence that developmentally early bodily experience is foundational for all kinds of thought, including the capacity for abstract reasoning and conceptualization. The body is the foundation for the mind because it is the primary spatial and temporal interactions of bodies with their surroundings (perception, movement, and actions) that assemble the structures for thought: first a wordless awareness of the body's perceptions and acts, and eventually the structures of conscious and symbolic thought. But the level of wordless awareness persists as the organizing principle of most of the body's everyday being-in-the-world. In suggesting that cognitive capacities are, in a sense, the spin-offs of accumulated bodily spatiotemporal actions in the material world, Merleau-Ponty is led to conclude that the body is the foundation of imaginative and analytical processes as well: that the embodied, nonconceptual content of experience underlies all our subsequent categories, priorities, and judgments.

For Merleau-Ponty, mind is the activity of a body that is engaged in spatial and temporal relations with other objects and people. He later moved on from applying this solely to perception as a mode of thought, to the nature of linguistic and social communication in general. This later work, influenced by Saussurian linguistics, looked at how signs and symbols transport cognition beyond the world of immediate perception. But to Merleau-Ponty even words are an embodied phenomenon: "What remains to me of the word once learnt is its style as constituted by its formation and sound. . . . I possess its articulatory and acoustic style as one of the modulations, one of the possible uses of my body" (Merleau-Ponty 2002, 209–10).

Corporeal Schema

Merleau-Ponty used the notion of the corporeal or body schema to describe the prereflexive sense of the boundaries of the subject's body and what it and its constituent parts are doing. It's this proprioception that tells us where we end and everything else begins (even if in reality that boundary is not always as sharp as we think). It enables us to move and position ourselves without having consciously to think about it, except in aberrational circumstances when the schema is disrupted through brain trauma, illness, or drugs. Both psychoanalysis and developmental neurology theorize that the sense of boundedness and bodily self-control that emerges in early life is linked to the parallel emergence of an integrated psychic sense of self. Before and for a while after birth it seems likely that an infant does not possess much of a self/other boundary in terms of its sensations, structures, orientation to other objects, and so on. A coherent somatic and psychic identity is acquired painstakingly, through the repetition of bodily actions, as initially fragmented perceptions coalesce into a more or less stable sense of more or less self-controlled separateness from other animate and inanimate objects.[3]

The idea of the corporeal schema, assembled through the organization of tactile, kinesthetic, and proprioceptive inputs, has reemerged in contemporary neuroscientific work on embodiment, where it is more usually referred to as *body schema*. I will be returning to current cognitive science in a moment, but for now want only to highlight the body schema as a bridging concept between the older philosophical phenomenology of Merleau-Ponty and twenty-first century neuroscience. The scientific literature differentiates between the corporeal, or *body schema*, a set of sensorimotor processes that operate below the level of awareness, and the *body image*, a culturally derived and usually conscious system of perceptions, concepts, and beliefs about one's body.[4] Making sense of the psychological, clinical, cognitive scientific, and philosophical literature on embodiment and cognition is not helped by the fact that these two terms, and others,[5] are defined and used variously in different disciplines. For our purposes, I want to keep body image and body schema as conceptually separated as possible (acknowledging that rigid separation at times is artificial), because body image and body schema will be differently affected by cultural attitudes toward disability. The two can be distinguished in terms of their availability to consciousness. Body image is a set of beliefs and representations, the intentional object of which is the subject's body. As the conceptual understanding or emotional apprehension of the body, a person's own body image will be affected, for better or worse, by sociocultural beliefs about phenotypic variation. Because many aspects of body image are conscious and can be put into words, it is amenable to revision—a negative body image can be changed through conscious cognitive work.[6]

The body schema, on the other hand, lies outside of consciousness and operates below the level of the subject's intentionality (Gallagher and Cole 1995, 371). It is an interior construction that refers not just to how the body is, but how it is in relation to its surroundings. The schema therefore supports a dynamic, dialectical epistemology that dissolves the distinction of subject/object. Knowledge of the world and its object components is mediated through the corporeal expressions of action and competences, and these are in turn modified through repeated patterns of encounter with the world. As Gallagher puts it, "The mature operation of a body schema depends on a developed perceptual knowledge of one's own body: and the organized perception of one's own body, *and then of the external world*, depends on the proper functioning of the body schema" (Gallagher 2005, 67; my italics). If this is the case, then the corporeal schema can be seen as the vehicle for the physical and mental dispositions that Bourdieu talks about, that facilitate our acting without having to think about it and things appearing to us, perceptually and semantically, as they do.

THE EMBODIED MIND IN COGNITIVE SCIENCE

In discussing the corporeal schema I introduced some ideas of contemporary cognitive science. These ideas become necessary at this point because, although Merleau-Ponty makes a persuasive *phenomenological* case for the embodiment of mind, those wanting the explanatory dots to join up will be left unsatisfied. As a philosopher and not a physiologist, Merleau-Ponty does not take up the question of what sort of mechanism might possibly transform primary sensorimotor experience into higher-order thinking. This is true even though, unlike his phenomenological contemporaries, he draws extensively on existing psychological, psychoanalytic, and, most significantly, neurophysiological studies to support his philosophical arguments about cognition. Much of his empirical data comes from neuropathology because the effects of disruptions to the standard sensory and motor apparatus were useful in his philosophical modeling of phenomenological norms. In his later work[7] he is concerned that conceptual forms of knowing acknowledge their dependence on and origins in perception, and he turns his attention to describing the elaboration of higher-order cognition, especially communication with others, through and beyond perception (Merleau-Ponty 1964; Sallis 1981). But largely because of the limits to the neurological knowledge of his time, Merleau-Ponty cannot propose a process through which embodiment might determine significant aspects of complex cognition. While the elaboration of an embodied basis for primary consciousness might be plausible, it is harder to connect this to the development of symbolic thinking, conceptualization, imagination, memory, and so on.

Because of this, it is difficult to make informed suggestions about what kind of difference an *anomalous body* might make to higher-order cognition. We could predict that not having standard-issue arms and legs, for instance, will result in an unusual orientation of body to surroundings, establishing and reinforcing slightly variant pathways of sensory input and motor response, and in Merleau-Ponty's phenomenology this would matter for the subject's grip on the world—indeed, whether it is possible to establish an adequate grip at all. But to suggest that this might influence the complex processes of abstract thought seems a bit more of a jump.

Embodied Cognition

Over the last couple of decades, support for a so-called embodied cognition has been gaining ground within neuroscience. Embodied cognition claims that complex mental processes are founded on the physical interactions that people have with their environment;[8] this is contrasted with the classic or first-generation view of cognition as essentially computational and rule based. In the next part of this chapter I focus on the theoretical framework of embodied cognition, not because it is necessarily correct, or the best one for understanding the relationship of anomalous body to thought, but because I think it is important to show that there are models for thinking through how having/being an anomalous embodiment may contribute to distinct moral understandings. With models and mechanisms at hand, empirical investigation becomes possible.

A diversity of views on embodied cognition exist, and a comprehensive review of them and of their implications for theorizing ethics in disability is beyond what I can do here.[9] Behind all of them is the idea, familiar from Merleau-Ponty's phenomenology, that a subject's sensorimotor capacities and the environment in which they operate combine to facilitate the development of specific cognitive capacities. Early subjective experience of the body interacting with the material world generates neural substrates, which are then available to form the basis for thought and later language. Humans and other primates are born with the basics of a distributed neural network.[10] This is developmentally refined through "systematic interactions between tactile, proprioceptive and vestibular inputs, as well as between such inputs and the visual perception of the structure and movements of one's own and other people's bodies" (Berlucchi and Aglioti 1997, 560), which is how cognitive scientists describe what babies and infants do (Thelen 1995; Thelen and Smith 1994).

Hence cognition emerges from constraints that are both intrinsic (to the neural substrate) and environmental (Westermann et al. 2006). This is a radical break from the view of cognition and consciousness that prevailed in mid- to late-twentieth century cognitive science, in which a subject's mental events operate pretty much independently of the organic matter, other than neural tissue, of which the subject is composed. (It's on the basis of this view of consciousness that some proponents of trans- or post-humanism look forward to the day when personal identity, by which they tend to mean cognition, can be uploaded onto an informational matrix.)

Embodied Language

In the embodied cognition thesis, data from a range of cognitive science subdisciplines come together to support the general hypothesis that aspects of bodily experience are used to structure abstract concepts. But if the structures that support cognition cantilever out from more basic neural structures (Westermann et al. 2006), that still leaves the question of how exactly that get us from bodies to moral thinking. As examples, I outline two approaches to embodied cognition that have strong implications for embodied moral understanding. One of these is the view that abstract concepts (including moral ones such as "autonomy" and "justice") are understood through embodied metaphor. The second approach links moral evaluation to the body through embodied emotion.

Embodied Metaphor

Cognitive linguists have long puzzled over the human capacity to understand and use abstract concepts such as those deployed in moral discourse. Although linguistics has traditionally treated language as an abstract propositional system independent of embodiment, new lines of work present a case for the view that the body, or more precisely the body's sensory and motor experience, has something to do with how people understand certain words and phrases, and how these words and phrases, and not others, emerge in language to carry their meanings. In this view, conceptual abstraction is not primarily mediated through representations and propositions, but through embodied interactions, especially patterns of bodily actions, perceptions, and manipulations of objects (Lakoff and Johnson 1980, 1999, 2002; Johnson 1987; Gibbs 1996). Briefly, the idea is that in the course of interacting habitually with the world and objects in it, what are called image schemas are generated. Despite their name, *image schemas* are not mental pictures. They are a hypothetical combination of visual, auditory, tactile, and kinesthetic components in "experiential gestalts" (Gibbs et al. 2004, 1192) that give coherence to recurring perceptual and motor bodily experiences. An example that appears in the literature here is that of an image schema for *balance* (Gibbs 2005; Johnson 1987). Early physical experiences of balance and disequilibrium, ranging from the obvious (losing one's balance and falling over) to the less so (feeling too cold or too hot, too wet or too dry) give us, it is supposed, a felt sense of the meaning of being in balance or being unbalanced.

Image schematic structuring is proposed to lie at the heart of the capacity to symbolize and conceptualize. Image schemata provide a bundled-up, generalizable sense of one cluster of experience which can then be systematically associated with other clusters (Gibbs and Colston 1995). Mapping

one domain to another, related one is effectively a process of metaphor construction. The key point here is that conceptual metaphors can associate a
concrete source domain with an abstract target domain.[11] An image schema
to do with verticality, deriving from the human experience of acquiring upright posture, links uprightness with abstractions of elevated power and status, and this is revealed linguistically in the use of metaphorical phrases: to
look up to, or to be *high born* (Gibbs 1992; Gibbs and Steen 1999). A schema
stemming from our experiences of containing (or all too often, in early experience, failing to contain) bodily contents, or of being contained by other
persons or objects, allows us to conceptualize not only material insides and
outsides, and volumes and spaces, but also the bounding of abstract entities such as the self, an academic discipline, the mind, a nation or culture,
or an emotion (Johnson 1987; Gibbs 2003). Moreover, people make sense
of the many different (literal and metaphorical) uses of a polysemous word
like *stand* because the everyday bodily experience of standing gives rise to
multiple image schemas that ground people's understanding of the various
physical meanings of stand, but also its metaphorical uses (to take a stand
on an issue, to stand for something, and so on) (Gibbs et al. 1994). The
proponents of this model say that the ready availability of image schemata
for metaphorical concepts makes possible the fluid mental manipulation of
complex thought.

The claim here is that we understand the nonliteral meanings of metaphors
not because they are linguistic conventions that we have picked up, but because they have embodied meaning for us. There is substantiating psycholin-
guistic evidence that embodied experience connects with, and can even be
used to predict, the use of particular idioms (Gibbs 1992, 2003). Data from
these experiments are interpreted to mean that the way in which people understand a given fundamental body experience (these experiments used the
experience of hunger) predicts which concepts of the source domain they will
draw on when talking or writing about a related abstract concept (in the case
of hunger, the related concepts of desire or need). I want to emphasize here
that these theorists do not claim that the body is *all there is* for cognition; social organizations and culture provide additional frames and constraints, and
embodied associations are to an extent culturally modifiable. When students
in the United States and Brazil were compared to see how the concepts of
"hunger" and "thirst" were used to describe metaphorically other experiences
of desire (he thirsts for revenge, she hungers for power), it is true there was re-
markable consistency in the way language was used and in which metaphorical extrapolations were found to be appropriate. But there were also some
variations which the authors took as indicating the impact of socially distinct
experiences: poverty, and the everyday experience of chronic hunger rather
than occasional peckishness, being a lived reality to more of the Brazilian students than to those from California (Gibbs et al. 2004).

The embodied metaphor thesis is not universally accepted by cognitive linguists. Critics say that the available evidence simply does not yet allow us to distinguish a model in which sensorimotor experience is foundational to the understanding of abstract concepts from one in which the association between particular spatial relationships and those concepts is purely conventional and learned (Murphy 1996; Glucksberg 2001). But *if* it really is the case that people use aspects of their phenomenal experience to structure abstract concepts, then the experiential elements connected to concepts (the connection of verticality to dominance, or of balance to fairness) are irreducible parts of our core understanding of them.

Embodied Moral Emotion

An alternative route by which the experience of the body could "get into" or underpin higher-order cognition, and especially moral thinking, is through the embodiment of particular emotional states rather than language or conceptualization. This proposal is particularly interesting because not only is it more intuitively graspable than models dealing in cognitive linguistics; it is also consistent with recent neurocognitive studies confirming the role of emotion in everyday moral responses (Greene et al. 2001; Greene and Haidt 2002; Moll et al. 2002). Neuroimaging techniques suggest that as experimental subjects perform moral-reasoning tasks, areas in the brain known to be involved in emotional responses become more metabolically active, and there is also evidence that different types of moral transgression consistently elicit certain emotional responses (Rozin et al. 1999; Shweder et al. 1997). Some theorists conclude from this that our response to morally loaded events is based on the emotions they stir up in us, or the memory of what we felt on analogous occasions in the past. This applies at least to our initial response, our "gut reaction," whatever more reasoned processes are applied later (Haidt 2001). The moral concepts of "good" and "bad" become in this Humean view the perceptual-motor records of dispositions to experience emotions on particular occasions that are, at their most primitive, to do with good and bad sensations. Jesse Prinz (2005) suggests that basic moral concepts like good, bad, justice, truth, duty, responsibility, entitlement, together with concepts that have moral dimensions like courage, ownership, or care, are constituted through patterns of practices and their associated emotions. Prinz suggests that our grasp of the concept of ownership, and the moral concepts associated with it, is rooted in the emotions associated with the practices of ownership (satisfaction, frustration, jealousy, and so on). This is a quite different approach from that of the cognitive linguists, who would suggest that the morally congruent aspects of ownership are elaborated from the sensorimotor experiences of (for example) holding or grasping a possession.

THE PLACE OF VARIANT BODIES

From the perspective of disability, the truly striking thing about both phenomenological and neuroscientific theories is the virtually exclusive focus
on normative forms of embodiment. Despite his status in Western philosophy as "something like the patron saint of the body" (Shusterman 2005,
151), Merleau-Ponty said almost nothing about body forms that are
nonnormative by virtue of not being male. Even his writing on sexuality, a
topic which clearly has *something* to do with gendered difference, takes as
standard the male embodied experience. Feminist phenomenologists have
severely criticized his work for this neglect. Iris Marion Young notes that Merleau-Ponty simply fails to provide any account of the forms of corporeality
that are specific to women, such as the gendered experiences of pregnancy or
having breasts (Young 2005), while even more damningly, according to Elizabeth Grosz, "Never once in his writings does he make any suggestion that
his formulations may have been derived from the valorization and analysis
of the experience of only one kind of subject. The question of what other
types of human experience, what other modalities of perception, what other
relations subjects may have with objects is not, cannot be, raised in the terms
he develops" (Grosz 1994, 110). Ultimately Merleau-Ponty and—less for-
givably—later phenomenologists ignore or write off as marginal any experiences of corporeality that are not those of the male standard.

Criticism of phenomenology's neglect of the gendered body applies
equally well to its treatment of other types of phenotypic variance. Certainly, Merleau-Ponty occasionally engages with impaired embodiment in
brief discussions of visual impairment in the context of extensions to the
corporeal schema. He uses neuropathological data, like the case of the
brain-damaged Schneider (Merleau-Ponty 2002, 118–59), to explore some
of the consequences of anomalies in perception and neural integration,
and he refers to the effect of illness, saying that in disease states the body's
intentional arc "goes limp" (157). But these are all references to illness as
a disruption or breakdown of the unified lived body (Diprose 1994, 106);
they are not about a different kind of body having a different kind of corporeal schema, one that is as normal and functional to that subject as the
"normal" body is to others. Perhaps it is that the commitment to establishing a universal phenomenological ontology renders Merleau-Ponty
and other phenomenologists incapable of acknowledging any variation in
the primary normative experience that might challenge the claim that
being-in-the-world can be described in terms of a common primordial perception.

But a phenomenology that splits the experience of being-in-the-world
into the normal (the one we focus on) and the pathological (variants that
are interesting only for what they tell us about normality) obscures the very

obvious fact that even fully functioning people vary enormously in their capacity for certain perceptions or actions that, in principle, all human beings are supposed to be able to do. Whenever the "normal" spontaneous body sense is invoked, we need to keep in mind that this sense operates along something like a continuum with multiple axes. Even in "normal" people, the intentional arc of perception and motion that Merleau-Ponty takes as universal and foundational to thinking is often, in reality, awkward, incomplete, or flawed. Irrespective of the amount of practice, some of us will always drop the ball; others will always have two left feet when it comes to the tango. In body phenomenology not much attention has been paid to such variation, nor to the extremes that shade toward the anomalous at both ends of the spectrum of competence.

And currently at least, cognitive science is also vulnerable at this point. The data I sketched out previously come from experiments and observations using nondisabled people as experimental subjects. I am not aware of any studies carried out within the embodied cognition paradigm that have tried specifically to take into account differences in perceptual and motor experiences that follow from having a body that senses or moves in a different way from the norm. This is a significant gap since, according to the embodied mind paradigm, it's the *particularities* of an organism's embodiment that largely determine the nature of the experiences that serve as its basis for cognition. If sensorimotor experiences shape the conceptual categories that we are able to construct, they also, in the end, shape how the world appears to us, and the paradigm suggests that changing the particularities of the body would have some effect on cognition. There are one or two brief comments in the literature that point to it in principle as a possible source of variation. Van Rompay et al. (2005), for instance, comment that "the embodied interactions of a handicapped person differ substantially from the interactions of those fully mobile." These aside, cognitive scientists, like most phenomenologists, have not yet acknowledged that the body of their subject does not necessarily adhere to a universal human form.

Ironically, more consideration has been given to the effect on the corporeal schema of the body's habitual association with objects such as tools, clothes, vehicles, or jewelry. This also has special resonance for disabled people, many of whom live in long-term association with different assistive devices: canes, wheelchairs, prosthetic limbs, hearing aids, or guide dogs. Experimental psychology and clinical neurobiology have both provided compelling evidence that body schemas can morph to continuously reconfigure the individual's state of being-in-the-world and to include objects that are not organically part of the body. And Merleau-Ponty himself maintained that the body is *not* defined by the boundary of the skin, but extends itself by rendering some external objects as within those boundaries. The

corporeal schema is in constant flux to incorporate some and separate off
other specific external objects:

> If I am in the habit of driving a car, I enter a narrow opening and see that I can't
> "get through" without comparing the width of the opening with that of the wings,
> just as I go through a doorway without checking the width of the doorway against
> that of my body. The car has ceased to be an object. . . . The blind man's stick has
> ceased to be an object for him, and is no longer perceived for itself; its point has
> become an area of sensitivity, extending the scope and active radius of touch, and
> providing a parallel to sight. In the exploration of things, the length of the stick
> does not enter expressly as a middle term: the blind man is rather aware of it
> through the position of objects than of the position of objects through it. . . . To
> get used to . . . a stick, is to be transplanted into [it], or conversely, to incorporate
> [it] into the bulk of our own bodies (Merleau-Ponty 2002, 165–66)

Recent work with neuroprosthetic limbs confirms that interaction with external objects prompts some rewiring of neural connectivity. More strik-
ingly, it also suggests that the external object need not even be in physical
contact with the body. A group working at Duke University has reported
that macaque and rhesus monkeys could learn to control *unattached* robotic
arms by means of brain signals alone, using a brain-machine interface.[12] In
May 2005 it was reported that these monkeys showed remodeling of the
neural circuits that were used to control their own, attached arms. Neuronal
connections appeared to have been shifted to enable the monkey's brain to
incorporate properties of the robotic arm as if it were another arm. The in-
vestigators argued that these results extend the accepted view of brain plasticity to include prosthetics of various kinds: "Everything from cars to clothing that we use in our lives becomes incorporated into our sense of self."[13]

Quite how far this can be taken, and especially whether it can be extended
to such "objects" as assistive animals or other persons, are the next questions—unanswerable at present because of the lack of data. There are scat-
tered and tantalizing hints from different areas, perhaps most intriguingly
from subjective accounts of prosthetic use. A fascinating example is given in
the anthropologist Gelya Frank's long-term study of a woman, Diane De-
Vries, who like Alison Lapper was born with vestigial limbs. Frank writes:

> Many of the experiences Diane eventually described did not fit neatly within
> the conventional concept of the "body." For example, Diane's interdependence
> with others . . . engendered an intimacy and identification that defied normal
> definitions of the bounded body. Consider Diane's participation in [her sister
> Debbie's] learning to dance: "It's true that there is a Diane within this Diane
> who can dance, which enabled me to teach my younger sister Debbie. But
> there's another reason I could coach her so well. [I not only saw her body mov-
> ing,] I felt her movements in a sense, part of her body (the part I lacked on the
> exterior) was mine too. So, since I knew how her body moved, I could coach
> her in dancing." (Frank 2000, 124)

If it is true that pervasive sensory and motor pathways are what give the basic framework for consciousness, and that body experiences generate image schemas that underpin a host of related concrete and abstract concepts, one prediction would be that where those basic pathways differ as a result of different sensorimotor input, the resulting cognitive processes are not going to be identical either. As a result, phenotypic variation might have unanticipated effects on cognitive processes. Of course, other outcomes are equally possible. It could be that the magnitude of difference may be too minor to have a discernible effect, or that the high degree of plasticity and/or redundancy that is so often observed in neural and biological processes ensures that in practice, altered sensorimotor inputs are channelled into common conserved pathways so that the end result, in terms of cognition, is indistinguishable from the norm. At the moment, with the present level of neuroscientific understanding and lack of empirical data, we are simply not in a position to make much of a guess of how much, or what kind, of difference it might make.

Taken to its extreme, the argument that perceptual and motor intentionality are involved in building the cognitive structures for reflective and discursive thought would predict that a person who, for example, was unable from birth to make voluntary, repeated bodily actions would also end up unable to *think* (or at least to think anything like others do). And this is obvious nonsense. Even given that such impairments are uncommon, there is not a vestige of empirical or anecdotal evidence to back up such a strong conclusion. People who from birth have a severely compromised capacity for self-controlled movement, perhaps as a result of cerebral palsy or hereditary myopathies, as a general rule are absolutely cognitively intact. More plausible is the weaker claim that the corporeal schema of, say, a person with congenital limb anomalies or other kinds of skeletal dysplasia, a conjoined twin, or a lifelong wheelchair user will be different in some significant ways from the corporeal schema of a person with a standard body. Whether and to what extent this is true for people with less physically extensive impairments, which have less impact on gross morphology or motor ability, is not a question we can answer at the moment. At first glance, I find it intuitively unlikely that minor variations—congenital deafness, for example, or ectrodactyly[14]—could significantly alter a subject's body schema. And yet if I think about personal experience (an empirical sample of n = 1), I know from video evidence and from what friends have told me that I orient myself constantly with reference to the sources of sound, and more importantly for me, light, in ways that are subtly unlike the ways of hearing people. I'm certainly not conscious of doing it, but it suggests that my perceptual and motor organization is responding to environmental cues and working with them differently than it does for audionormals.

What about the effects of modified body-environment interactions on higher-order cognition? According to Mark Johnson, one of the first philosophers to take neurolinguistic work into the context of ethics, the embodied construction of conceptual metaphor has profound ethical implications. In his book on moral imagination, Johnson (1993) suggests that everyday *moral* thinking is organized through metaphors and semantic frames ultimately rooted in bodily processes. Under moral thinking he includes a range of processes from the description of moral situations to the analytical thinking that leads to moral evaluations, judgments, and fundamental moral abstractions (freedom, duties, rights, action). Rights, for instance, are seen as possessions (I have this right; you owe me that as a right). Duties are burdens (his duties weigh him down; can we take some of the load off?). Rights and responsibilities should be in equilibrium (with rights come responsibility). In the embodied metaphor model, image schemata about verticality and balance generate foundational ideas about the moral worth of balance and equilibrium. The reflection of this in everyday moral discourse is that we then speak approvingly about a *balance of power*, or a *well-balanced* argument or person; fairness is about being *even handed*; political and intellectual *instability* is to be avoided. Similarly, the embodied value given to being vertical and upright, higher rather than lower, is transferred to the moral domain metaphorically through corresponding phrases: thus a good man is an *upright person*, or *high minded*; or conversely, *falls* from grace. Someone can *stand on her own two feet*, or conversely has to be *carried by everyone else*. Social policies ensure that people are *lifted out of* poverty.

Metaphors or other linguistic devices, which are often assumed to be understood in the same way by everyone with a shared cultural background, may then have subtly different resonances for different embodied minds. Because I am visually biased, the phrase "I see what you mean," commonly used for the act of understanding someone's speech, is one I use rather comfortably. On the other hand, "I hear what you're saying," used to connote deeper empathy, the act of going beneath the words to get the implied message, is a phrase with which I never have felt at ease. And on examining this response I find that in part it is because that phrase is phenomenologically impoverished for me. While I generally see the meaning in words, meaning is less easily conveyed to me aurally. It is also because my experience of auditory meaning is not absent, but qualitatively *different*: to me, "I hear what you're saying" does not convey a sense of grasping a subtly delivered message, but rather an act of piecing together very fragmented information with the help of some nifty guesswork. In place of a message of deep perception and empathy, then, my use of this phrase has more to do with effort and the increased risk of misunderstanding.

The thesis of embodied *emotional* responses has other implications. Prinz (2005) says that moral concepts are derived from emotional responses to events and situations. These responses are likely to be a mixture of innate (all babies are upset and cry when startled) and learned (socialization teaches us to feel guilty for taking something that doesn't belong to us). Obviously there are impairments that directly affect perceptual or motor experience: a visually impaired baby will not startle at a sudden movement in its visual field. However, although visual impairment might have larger effects in other areas of life, it's hard to see how it would be a major impediment to the acquisition of a basic sense of good things and bad things, since any visually impaired infant with intact cognitive function will have enough alternative, nonvisual experiences to get the general idea about good and bad. Startling at a loud noise or cold air, for instance, will just as effectively convey a sense of what "unpleasant" means.

It might work otherwise, though, for more sophisticated moral concepts, such as equality, autonomy, selfishness, or responsibility. It's suggested that an understanding of these concepts derives from the emotional responses we have, and learn how to name, in particular situations that instantiate the concepts themselves. So, on an everyday level, the substantive content of "generosity" is picked up from distinctive patterns of behaviors (freely giving something, holding it back, asking for something) and the patterns of emotions (pleasure, anger, frustration) that are associated with those behaviors. With this model, then, a disabled person could experience significantly different *patterns of behaviors* (enacted between herself and other people) and hence experience emotional responses unlike those of nondisabled people. As one example: many disabled children are subjected to unasked-for encroachment on their physical integrity through medical procedures or physiotherapy, or simply because of communication barriers, of a different type and at a later age than nondisabled children. As nondisabled children grow up they are guided by parents and teachers to associate unwanted physical intrusions with a sense of affront or outrage and to name it as abuse. But for some disabled children there will be neither encouragement nor opportunity to do so, and so they may not come to share the understanding of these acts as morally reprehensible. There is evidence for this: in Shakespeare, Gillespie-Sells, and Davies' study of disabled sexuality, a woman with polio is quoted as saying how sexual abuse "just seemed the same as everything else that had been done to me. . . . What the doctors did, they lifted up my night-dress, they poked here and they pushed here without asking me. . . . I didn't say no to any doctor [so] the porter actually was to me doing absolutely nothing different at all than every doctor or nurse had ever done" (Westcott 1993, 17, quoted in Shakespeare et al. 1996, 142).

The generation of moral understandings through emotional linkage to embodied practices brings us quite close to Bourdieu's proposal that the tacit rules for social practices are incorporated into a habitus of preconscious dispositions to evaluate and categorize. In terms of embodied emotion much the same idea is placed in a cognitive framework, tracing moral responses back to habits of behavior and affect.

IMPLICATIONS

All of this has some interesting implications. The embodied mind and conceptual metaphor theses broadly suggest that in everyday moral thinking, any situation, including situations of moral difficulty, will be conceptualized predominantly through shared metaphors, semantic frames, or narrative structures. Insofar as these include moral concepts, it would mean that our preexisting embodied judgments of the morally relevant features of the situation are applied in the very act of describing it. The unreflective use of metaphors (or narrative structures, as we will see in the next chapter) in our descriptive and analytical work with moral issues will condition the kind of reasoning we can do about them and the conclusions we can reach. It is important to be aware of this possibility in general because, in order to be properly alert to the distorting effects of bias, we need to recognize the conceptual frameworks inherited from our social and moral tradition, or our embodied experience. It also helps to grasp that the same situation can be framed differently according to the choices of metaphor, while different sets of metaphors will have different moral obligations arising from them. Bioethics is becoming more comfortable these days with the idea that social position has an influence on the way a person describes an event, issue, or quandary. The less-familiar idea is that the biophysical, as well as social, nature of a person's embodied presence in the world also exerts an effect on moral perception and interpretation. Through Merleau-Ponty's primary "silent consciousness" and the newer paradigm of embodied cognition, it becomes possible to imagine how particular body shapes, movements, and practices take on the felt status of normality. These theories of embodied cognition and cognitive linguistics, then, enable us to propose, even tentatively, mechanisms by which the normative force of specific perceptual or motor experiences lines up behind concepts and linguistic constructions. The embodied, preconsciously encoded nature of these dispositions makes them virtually unassailable, at least until presented with an external challenge, such as phenotypic anomaly.

A second consequence is that people who, because of their impairments, fail to embody certain valued metaphors—are not upright, cannot stand on their own two feet, lack get-up-and-go, and so on—will not be afforded the positive connotations that go along with the approved terms. Of course, these associations are not made consciously, and the vocabulary is not (or very rarely) chosen deliberately to set particular meanings to work. But as I discussed in chapter 2, the unconscious layers of meaning contained within certain words or phrases are potent. In everyday discourse, more of our terminology than we realize carries unspoken statements about our own or others' moral status or competence. Kay Toombs understands this when she says, writing about chronic illness, that "the value assigned to upright posture should not be underestimated. . . . Verticality is directly related to autonomy. Just as the infant's sense of autonomy and independence are enhanced by the development of the ability to maintain an upright posture . . . so there is a corresponding loss of autonomy which accompanies the loss of uprightness" (Toombs 1993, 65).

The point of greatest relevance to disability ethics, as opposed to the ethics of disability, is this: if it can be shown that bodies with qualitatively unusual interactions with the material world generate subtly different structures of meaning, we have to consider seriously the possibility that having/being an anomalous embodiment might shape the language and concepts that build moral understanding. Every form of morally relevant thinking would be touched by this, from everyday speech to the technicalities of ethical theory, the use of metaphor to align description with moral intuitions, and the substantive content of basic ethical concepts. It is necessary to emphasize this last point because it is not just the habitual, loose, everyday sort of moral cognition that would be shot through with such bodily recollection. Professional bioethical discourse cannot consider itself, as the metaphor would put it, above all that. Academic ethics relies on rigorously crafted definitions of concepts like autonomy, independence, obligation, dignity, and freedom, which are the currency of the discipline. Feminist ethical theory has long criticized the traditional framings of such terms as inadequate because they are *idealized*, that is, failing to do necessary justice to the real ethical life of anyone in real societies; and inadequate because they are *gendered*, in that they also fail to reflect that women may have different understandings of those same concepts because their experiences may be different from those of men. And many feminist ethicists have been careful to acknowledge that the exclusion of gendered knowledge is one case of a broader exclusion of marginal epistemologies. What needs more exploration here is the distinctive contribution of embodied difference to moral epistemology. By this I mean looking out for those aspects of moral understanding which are molded not only by social positioning, but also through the body and its neurophysiological mediation of difference.

This is the marginality of people whose embodied experience calls into question the common understanding of moral terms. So if "balance" were experientially understood as something achieved only imperfectly, or maintained by overshooting the balance point and correcting, or accomplished only with the help of other people or assistive devices, then discussions about "the balance of nature," "balancing rights," or even what is entailed in best-practice "reflective equilibrium" might take quite different forms.

Or to take another idea that is commonly pulled into the discussion of autonomy and self-determination: the self as a defined unit. When we use expressions like "he is very self-contained," "she keeps herself to herself," or alternatively, "he's all over the place," and so on, we are mobilizing a set of associations that color our conceptualization of identity and self-control. If the self is a container, then its contents define the nature of the self. The more firmly contained, the more of a distinct self it is, and the better able to make decisions for itself. The "naturalness" of the self-is-a-container metaphor comes from the lifelong subjective experience of our psychic and somatic integrity—that which is at play when we exercise our autonomy—being bounded by the skin. But there are types of phenotypic variation that challenge these assumptions about the somatic boundaries of the self. The most extreme example of such a challenge is undoubtedly provided by conjoined twins. In her book on body anomaly, *One of Us*, Alice Dreger comprehensively demonstrates from the medical literature and her own research that when both conjoined twins are equivalently developed, the selves within the skin are separate, subjectively and objectively, despite the body's having a single boundary. Like nonconjoined people, conjoined twins experience themselves as independent individuals. "They do not think they need a discrete body to achieve independent status" (Dreger 2004, 32). Nonconjoined people, however, have their own beliefs about what it is like to live conjoined. They assume that it inevitably entails severe constraint and limitation, and this is reflected in the routine separation of conjoined twins surgically if it is possible to do so without killing them. Yet Dreger writes that "across cultures and across time, the great majority of people who are conjoined simply have not expressed the sensation of being overly confined, horribly dependent, physically trapped, or unwillingly chained to others" (32). What is true is that the nonconjoined majority of us will have experienced being able to exert control over our lives and being treated as decision-making individuals by others, in parallel with physically separating from our caregivers and doing more and more things "by ourselves." So it is not surprising that most of us have a strong intuition that being an autonomous moral agent goes along with having a somatic boundary that contains within it a single functioning self (4). The interesting question for disability bioethics is, exactly how would ethical discussions about the moral agent and agency, autonomy, dependence, and so on be altered, if they had to include the points of view of those who do not, either rationally or viscerally, share that intuition?

It is worth reiterating that my argument is *not* that having/being an unusual embodiment means that phenotypically variant people then go on to develop completely unique frameworks of understanding, incommensurable with those of "normal people." Nor does it mean that everything worth saying about disability ethics can be boiled down to a side effect of biological body difference. As we found out in chapter 2, separating out the effects *of* impairment and the effects of the social and cultural response *to* impairment is often neither practical nor politically desirable, but more importantly, it may not reflect the truth of what is going on either. Suppose it really is the case that prereflective moral cognition is mediated through sensorimotor pathways laid down by the body interacting with the environment, and that this happens differently when anomalous interactions are involved. It would still be true that adaptations of the environment are as distinctively formative of moral cognition as unusual morphologies, movements, or perceptions themselves. It certainly cannot lead to the essentialist conclusion that there is a "disability brain" or "disability mind" that is unlike, or should be treated as unlike, the brains of "normal people."

When we look at the place of bodies in classical phenomenology and conventional cognitive science, two things stand out. The first is that these disciplines, in principle, offer valuable conceptual spaces for rethinking phenotypic variation and moral cognition. The second is that in practice there is a lack of genuine theoretical engagement with, and more especially empirical data about, phenotypic variation and disability. Differences in corporeal schema or conceptual metaphor due to impairment are, I believe, likely to play some role in the subjective experience of disability but are unlikely to be the most significant factors. I might be wrong, though. The current problem for bioethicists and others interested in following up on this is that however suggestive the models, the data just aren't there. Someone needs to go out and collect the phenomenological accounts, or do the neuroimaging, before we can tell how much houseroom to give to primary consciousness or embodied cognition in disability ethics.

Even if the original locus of meaning is the preconceptual bodily engagement with the world, this isn't an argument that it is or should be the only kind of cognition human beings engage in. Merleau-Ponty's contribution is to remind us, from within a tradition very different from feminist standpoint epistemology, that the rationalist philosophical view of the world "from nowhere" is always, in practice, the view from the body already immersed in the world it observes: a physical and social world that is both ontologically and epistemologically pervasive. Cognitive science's embodied mind provides more than one option for identifying the detailed and testable mechanisms by which the experience of disability can lead to modifications of moral perception and standpoint. Both phenomenological description and cognitive science are individualized approaches, and in this way they helpfully complement the more familiar perspectives of social epistemology. But because of this orientation, neither can adequately address the social, historical, economic, or political narratives within which bodies and behaviors are understood. That's the topic of the next chapter.

NOTES

1. So that *being-in-the-world* is something more like *being-in-the-body-in-the-world*.

2. In a lecture entitled "An End to Mediational Epistemology," November 2004, available at goodreads.ca/lectures/taylor/larkin-stuart04.html.

3. Note that Merleau-Ponty did not examine the possibility that the coherent sense of self might be a convenient fiction—something that the infant pulls together out of the chaos of impressions bombarding it in order to function at all, rather than a reflection of how things really are. Later, Lacan and others of the French psychoanalytic school did develop the idea of the self, or ego, as a cover for a truly fragmented psyche. Less attention has been given to the possibility that the sense of somatic unity is equally factitious.

4. Although Merleau-Ponty has been criticized for inconsistency in his use of terminology, Gallagher and Melzoff (1996) argue that in practice he does sustain a consistent distinction between *corporeal image* and *corporeal schema* throughout his work.

5. In addition to body image and body schema, some neuroscientists propose an interoceptive body sense associated with the internal autonomic system. Because it has less relevance to the differential interaction with the external world that I am suggesting for impairment, I do not discuss it further here. See also Craig (2002); De Preester (2007).

6. For example, in psychotherapies of patients with body dysmorphia.

7. Merleau-Ponty's final work, *The Visible and the Invisible* (1969), was left incomplete at his death.

8. For much more detail on embodied cognition and cognitive linguistics, see Pecher and Zwaan (2005), and Gallagher (2005).

9. See, for example, Wilson (2002), who identifies six distinct claims about embodied cognition: (1) cognition is situated, (2) cognition is time pressured, (3) cognitive work is off-loaded onto the environment, (4) the environment is part of the cognitive system, (5) cognition is connected with action, and (6) off-line cognition is body based—that is, sensorimotor functions that originally evolved to serve action and perception have been co-opted for use in the thought processes needed to think about situations and events in other times and places, that is, imagination and memory.

10. Just how much of it is inborn is a matter of dispute. There is debate over whether infants arrive in the world with no body image or schema (so that both are acquired as a result of postnatal experiences), or whether aspects of either image or schema are "innate"—genetic—or generated from very early prenatal experiences. This debate is well outside the scope of this book but can be followed in Gallagher (2005) and references therein. That at least something is present from the outset is supported by evidence that babies can imitate facial and bodily movements and expressions from very shortly after birth, and reports of phantom limb sensations in phocomelic children (that is, with congenital absence of limbs); see Thelen (1995), Thelen and Smith (1994), and Berlucchi and Aglioti (1997). Some work on embryonic development suggests that reflex movements begin as early as the seventh week of gestation, and there are some more controversial interpretations of behavioral

evidence for early self–nonself differentiation. As Gallagher drily notes, however, "Foetal phenomenology remains inaccessible."

11. For more details of this work see van Rompay et al. (2005) and Richardson et al. (2003).

12. Reported on the BBC online news service, October 13, 2003, at news.bbc .co.uk/2/hi/health/3186850.stm.

13. Reported on Duke University Pratt e-press, June 2005, at www.pratt.duke .edu/pratt_press/web.php?sid=230&iid=29.

14. The anomalous development of fingers and toes described in chapter 1.

6

Narratives of Disability: Models and Mentors

> To know who you are is to be oriented in moral space, a space in which questions arise about what is good or bad, what is worth doing and what not, what has meaning and importance for you and what is trivial and secondary.
>
> —Charles Taylor

> All our stories are about what happens to our wishes.
>
> —Adam Phillips

Meningitis is an inflammation of the meninges, the membrane around the brain. In the UK it kills around 150 children a year, despite the introduction of vaccination in 1998 (Enhanced Surveillance of Meningococcal Disease 2003). It is also the commonest cause of childhood sensorineural deafness, affecting about 15 percent of children who survive. At eight years of age I was sent home from the hospital with zero hearing in one ear and what would turn out to be a dying sputter in the other. My parents, grateful to have a live child to take home at all, did not at first grasp that a lot of my life was now radically different from before, and from anything they knew. It would now contain experiences they had never had (like having an ear mold fitted), and because virtually every moment of engagement with the world involved something that had to be done differently because hearing could not be a part of it, my life was altered on every front. The grandest themes of love, art, vocation, family, loyalty, revolutionary commitment, and so on, are ultimately constituted by the mundane details of whether you can understand the public announcements at the railway station en route to the barricades.

It was not that these things became impossible for me; it was that the hearing way of doing them became impossible. Neither my parents nor I had a clue about how to live as a deaf child. Like many others before me, I had to work out my own strategies for doing so.

As a result of the need for strategy I developed an obsession with literature about deafness. I read nonfiction, medical texts, autobiography, and all the novels there were, although the available fiction suggested my options were limited to becoming an art student before giving it all up for love of a hearing man *(The Day Is Ours,* Hilda Lewis), or a millworker and having hearing children who grew up to despise me *(In This Sign,* Joanna Greenberg). In common with many disabled adolescents who don't know adults with the same impairment, I was constantly in search of information about living with deafness that would instruct me in three central things: *This is how you do it, This is how you do it* _well_, and *This is who you are.*

A DISABILITY IDENTITY?

In the next two chapters, I look at aspects of what I will call "disability identity" and its moral significance. Identity today is a concept linking a broad range of concerns across disciplines, and any one of these disciplinary approaches would be illuminating. In this chapter, however, I focus on just one approach, narrative constructions of identities, and look at the role of disability memoirs in their *moral* construction. In the following chapter I shift from the personal to the political, to consider the ethical significance of political identification as a disabled person.

First some clarification of terms. The idea that each one of us has a unique, coherent, and continuing self-ness is fundamental to the contemporary way of making sense of the world (Gergen 1991; Harré 1991). Identity is invoked so often and so easily in both popular and academic discourse that it is easy to forget that the concept is dependent on specific background theories of how the sense of self is established and maintained. The word *identity* is also used with more than one meaning. For clarity's sake I try to distinguish between *self, identity,* and *subjectivity,* while acknowledging that the categories are overlapping, and that the way I use these terms is likely to be contested by other philosophers and neuroscientists interested in questions of personhood and consciousness. I'm simply going to acknowledge here that those debates exist, but will not enter into them.

So when I refer to the *sense of self* I mean the prelinguistic, somatic, and psychic sense we have of ourselves as unitary, bounded by skin and persistent over time. By *identity,* on the other hand, I mean the idea we have of ourselves as *particular* selves, the feeling that there are certain labels we would apply to ourselves and others we would disavow. My understanding of identity is broadly in line with those contemporary views that see it occupying the space where the somatic and psychic selves engage with and respond to the structures of the social world and with other people. Individual identity draws on features of the individual and from cultural resources that tell us which features are worth noticing, and what they signify. And by *subjectivity*, I mean the special understanding we have of ourselves as subjects of our lives, a sense of agency that arises out of the operation of our identities within the social world.

One way in which social understandings tell us who we are is through the categories of identity that are acknowledged and into which we are allocated. In terms of identification with a social or ontological organizational category—knowing what gender one is, which ethnicity, and so on—disabled people are anomalous in that they do not (usually) grow up surrounded by others like themselves, having their lives validated as normative. Unlike most ethnic minorities, a disabled person who wants to consider herself sharing a disability identity has to go and find the others before she can throw her lot in with them.

In fact, whether the concept of "disability identity" is analytically or practically helpful is a contested issue in disability studies. Some theorists argue vehemently for a singular disability identity, based on shared features such as the experience of oppression, and publicly enacted through the political disability movement. Others are equally convinced that invoking disability identity is essentializing something that is just too diverse, transient, and contingent to be so labelled (Price and Shildrick 1998; Corker 1999). I take up some of this debate when I return to the ethical consequences of a politics of recognition later on. Still, the discussion in the previous chapters suggested that phenotypic variation and the subjective experience of disability can affect how people perceive and make sense of their bodies, their surroundings, and the events of their lives. The sense that someone makes of her life is inextricably bound up with the person she thinks she is—her identity. Independent of whether we would want to claim there is some kind of shared or common disability identity, then, it seems plausible that impairment and impairment effects contribute to individual identity and subjectivity.

There is some empirical work in support of this. In the Swiss study I have already mentioned (Scully et al. 2004), we asked interview participants how they perceived the relationship between "their condition" and "their selves." Although the results can only be suggestive (exploring this issue was not the aim of the study overall and so we did not follow it up), they indicate that people with different impairments feel that it affects what they described as their identity, even when they did not accept the label of "disabled." However, the effect is not straightforward and certainly not uniform

across impairments. We had anticipated that there might be differences between the conditions we classed as "disabilities" (in the study these were
achondroplasia and hearing impairment) and as "chronic illnesses" (multiple sclerosis and cystic fibrosis), but it turned out the more significant distinction seemed to be between progressive and stable conditions. Almost
without exception our participants with skeletal dysplasia and hearing impairment agreed with the statement "my impairment is a part of me" and
for hearing impairment especially were likely to define it as "a positive part
of my identity." These participants were also relatively hostile to medical interventions that would remove the condition from themselves or from future generations. (Note, though, that all our hearing-impaired participants
had been deaf from birth or early childhood. Responses from people who
had lost their hearing in later life might well have been different.) By contrast, most participants with multiple sclerosis indicated it was "something
that has happened to me" or "a negative part of my identity"; none claimed
it as a positive part, and all of them were highly committed to the idea of
therapy or cure. The subjectivity of the person with MS must continually
adapt to changes in symptom severity, energy levels, capacities, and so on,
and it may be that such a process of repetitive loss prevents a current phenotypic state from being assimilated into a person's identity. While this is
also true for the person with cystic fibrosis, in this case the need for constant adaptation to changing health status has itself been part of the CF patient's experience from early childhood. Perhaps unsurprisingly, then, our
CF respondents were the most ambivalent of all participants toward their
illness and to the possibility of a cure. Nick Watson has some similar work,
in which he interprets his informants as overtly rejecting an identity based
on impairment ("I don't see myself as a disabled person"), while at the
same time integrating the impairment into their "ontological existence" but
in such a way as to "negate impairment as an identifier" (Watson 2002).

NARRATIVE IDENTITY

The "narrative turn" in psychology, sociology, and philosophy explores how
identities cohere around stories: those we are able to tell about ourselves,
and those others tell about us. As Somers (1994) notes, the narrative turn
is made possible by a shift from the traditional approach to narrative as a
representation of reality, toward a view of it as a constructive feature of social
epistemology and ontology. A constructionist approach to narrative sees it
as a key organizing principle, helping us to make sense of events and people. Some stories are told specifically to make *moral* sense, through identifying morally relevant features of the situation and locating them in a
framework of agreed normative concepts.

A narrative theory of identity says that stories, told by ourselves to our-selves, by ourselves to others, and by others to us, provide identities as well. Stories involve characters. They give a structure within which those characters' behavior makes sense. In one way or another they also tell us what our attitudes toward the characters and their acts should be. A con-structionist narrative approach to identity acknowledges that life and nar-rative are not the same, but neither are they separable: they are "part of the same fabric, in that life informs and is informed by stories" (Widders-hoven 1993, 2). According to narrative identity theorists, the process through which a personal identity is generated involves the ascription and the recognition of whole or part master narratives drawn from the cultural stock, and modified by the unique features of an individual life. The terms that I just defined as if they were separate (self, identity, subjectivity) are in reality ontologically and developmentally contiguous, as a human being moves from a primordial state of nondifferentiation to the recognition of the somatic and psychic self as separate, through conscious and uncon-scious identifications with other social beings, to an awareness of the self as part of a collective in which the "narratives of identity [are] embedded in other stories, including the wider stories of social and cultural settings" (Whitebrook 2001, 4). Narrative identity is both embodied and socially embedded.

At any historical moment, a culture lays claim to a finite repertoire of identity-forming stories, which fit the reality of some people's lives very well but of others' very poorly. This is why Hilde Lindemann Nelson and others argue that the process of narrative identity formation does not entail the uptake of a coherent unitary story, but rather the assembly of part-narratives that interweave through the flow of a life. Some narrative strands will be more prominent at certain times, others less so, and some may be abandoned altogether. The options available for individuals to "stitch to-gether satisfying identities" (Kenny 2004, 30) are limited by the cultural materials that are at hand. And except in the rare cases of the pathological liar or the analysand, assembling a self-constituting narrative is not gener-ally a conscious process. Nevertheless, there are times—perhaps through psychotherapy, as a result of a traumatic event, or through political cri-tique—when a person becomes acutely conscious of the *wrongness* of her current narrative of identity. While people who are unhappy with the way their life is going may try to change their circumstances or behavior, or even modify their values, people who are unhappy with their narrative of iden-tity have the task of finding a more satisfying story. The problem is that a "better" or the "right" story may be unavailable, or unavailable to them, in the time and culture to which they belong.

In focusing on narrative identity I am not making either the theoretical claim that identity is *only* explicable in terms of stories, or the methodological one that individual and collective identities are best understood through the narrative model. A full understanding of who we are depends on other things besides the story told. Narrative is not helpful in understanding the embodied, prelinguistic sense of self I described earlier, nor is narrative the best way to look at the desires and claims of a political group—although the political group, through its words and actions and existence, may reinforce or counteract a particular social narrative. But the narrative approach to identity helps to theorize how social formations and personal biography interact to give the sense of a meaningful identity and subjectivity. It has also raised a number of novel ethical questions, including what given narratives do to, for, and with people, and about the responsibility of communities to provide good narratives to live by.

THE MORAL SIGNIFICANCE OF NARRATIVE IDENTITY

The moral significance of identity narratives, and their master narratives, lies in their direct and indirect effects on a person's moral agency. Master narratives are encapsulations of what a society knows to be true about the right and wrong ways of being in the world. They describe model *types of people* (the teacher, the criminal, the student, the mother) as well as social or ontological *groups* (Muslims, white people, the middle class). As Lindemann Nelson points out (2001), master narratives are both explanatory and justificatory. They give emotionally and cognitively sound reasons, to ourselves and others, for what we do. In doing so, they justify our being the persons who do those things.

Because they are repositories of normative consensus, master narratives have enormous epistemological authority. They shape our moral imaginations. Once past what I call *first order recognition*, when we quickly categorize other people by gender, skin color, age, or body size and shape, we start to fit people into the broad narrative categories that go with those characteristics, usually well before we have the kind of data that would enable us to do this with real accuracy. Identifying a person as female immediately allocates her to a set of possible narratives (daughter, mother, dentist, Catholic) while making others a bit less likely (colonel, archbishop) and some impossible (sperm donor, pope). And because master narratives are generated within existing structures of domination and status, they have staying power as well, locked in place by the persistence of those structures.

Just because a collective narrative has epistemological authority, however, is no guarantee that it is epistemologically accurate, and its staying power does not prove it is morally praiseworthy. In *Damaged Identities, Narrative Repair*, Lindemann Nelson (2001) argues that many master narratives are in fact morally indefensible. Because the available narratives are generated and maintained within existing structures of power and domination, they will be constraining to all and actively oppressive to some. "Constraining to all" does not mean that everyone is constrained to the same degree or with the same result. The existence of master narratives within particular social arrangements means that no person has absolute freedom to assemble an identity; men as well as women, for instance, are limited in the narratives of identity they may adopt. Nevertheless, the number of master identities that are open for adoption, the degree of constraint the identity offers, and also how possible it is to resist the attribution of an unwanted identity or to take up a novel one, are markedly affected by other factors of social and political *Spielraum* and self-consciousness. Certain people have more of these than others.

TOXIC AND DAMAGING IDENTITIES

So narrative identities can be limiting, since there will be a finite number of them available and the parameters of story arc and character are more or less set. A *mother* narrative may not contain the option of hating one's off-spring, for example, so that a woman who finds herself in that position will "fall out of" the identity given by the narrative characteristics of mother. She is also likely to find there is no alternative narrative available (other than *bad mother*).

But as well as being limiting, narratives can also be morally untrustworthy. Lindemann Nelson focuses on what such narratives do to a person's moral agency via the effect on her identity. Identity is of fundamental importance to moral agency in part because our identities reflect the nature of the communities we inhabit, and hence the moral parameters within which we operate. Psychological and social identities also influence whether or not we can exercise agency at all. Lindemann Nelson sees having an "undamaged" identity as vital to moral agency, first because a person's freedom of action can be constrained through oppression by others who are taken in by the master narrative, and second, more subtly, through infiltration of a person's own consciousness so that he no longer believes himself to be capable of moral responsibility. When she writes that "freedom of agency requires not only certain capacities, competencies and intentions that lie within the individual, but also recognition on the part of others of *who one is*, morally speaking" (Lindemann Nelson 2001, 24), the first part of that sentence is about the limits to agency that accompany the internalization of a harmful identity that depletes a person's subjectivity. The second is about the kind of agency that others will allow a person with that identity to have, such as when a child with an impairment is considered ineducable and denied access to schooling, or when disabled people in general are not regarded as full members of civil society, so that no efforts are undertaken to make their participation more possible. Both processes interweave with each other, in that others' ascriptions form part of what is internalized, while self-belief will then generate patterns of behavior and response that others accept as characteristic of that kind of person.

Although in this chapter I concentrate on narrative as a whole, I don't want to forget that storytelling is a discursive process. Stories are put together from words, turns of phrase, descriptions, and metaphors, and these elements can individually be as powerfully toxic to the sense of subjectivity as the overall narrative sweep. Diana Tietjens Meyers holds that unconscious anxieties about otherness are stored in "culturally entrenched figurations" of certain social groups that allow prejudices to be transmitted and perpetuated (Meyers 1994, 44). Although some aspects of the discursive "figurations" of social groups can be changed by rational argument or through empirical data that run counter to harmful assumptions, Meyers is, I think, right to argue that what she calls "culturally normative prejudice" cannot be dismantled by "standard philosophical tactics" (44). The figurations she speaks of contribute to the narratives about the kinds of lives that we believe members of certain groups either *do* or *should* lead. And toxic stereotypes like these are not created through individual cognitive dysfunction or malice. They circulate culturally. As figurations in stories they have the ability to be transmitted "without obliging anyone [consciously] to formulate, accept or reject repugnant negative propositions about any group's standing or self-congratulatory positive propositions about one's own" (53). Fear, hatred, and contempt around marginalized entities and groups are perpetuated "behind 'is teeth," as my grandmother used to say, in metaphor and story line.

If individual narrative identities are assembled from elements of the larger stories available in our culture(s), and if identity underpins moral agency, then some master narratives cause moral damage. Their moral damage operates precisely through the distortion they cause to the cultural narratives about those persons and to the individual narratives of those concerned.

RECONSTRUCTIVE NARRATIVES

Both Lindemann Nelson and Meyers are suggesting that what is needed here is some form of discursive resistance, whether spontaneously arising in changing circumstances or consciously put together, that rejects the oppressive identity "and attempts to replace it with one that commands respect" (Lindemann Nelson 2001, 6). Where Meyers focuses more on a psychoanalytic methodology of bringing to consciousness the nonconscious or unconscious material and giving it benign expression through dissident speech of various kinds (Meyers 1994, 59), Lindemann Nelson undertakes discursive resistance through rewriting the story. At sites where social or cultural forces oppress through the shaping of narratives about particular kinds of people, so generating their own or others' expectations about moral competence, the *counterstories* identified by Lindemann Nelson reconfigure the narrative terrain about a group. They encourage self-understandings and the outsider's perceptions of members of a marginalized group to shift. Hence counterstories are potential channels for redefinition and moral transformation. The power of a master narrative to specify how members of marginalized groups, such as disabled people, are supposed to be depends on how widely it is accepted, and by whom (Lindemann Nelson 2001, 140). The efficacy of a counterstory, then, comes from its ability to disrupt the consensus around the dominant narratives and to suggest other possible lives.

What we have been talking about so far is the harm caused by figurative speech or narrative identities that limit the opportunities open to members of certain groups or that infiltrate their consciousness to compromise their moral agency. This applies to narrative identities that are present and are toxic. To this, however, I want to add another kind of problem. What happens when a narrative of identity is lacking? Not having a socially mandated identity at hand, even one that is oppressive and self-undermining (Appiah 2004, 191), is also damaging, although in a different ways. A person in this situation lacks a narrative pattern of life that matches the experiences she has or enables her to makes sense of her events and perceptions; lacks a language that enables her to name her experiences accurately and well and account for them to others; lacks a framework into which she can fit their choices and goals without distortion; lacks, at a most basic level, some of the templates for everyday living that the rest of us pick up from observation and from the stories we are told or read about or see on film.

In these cases, the words and life stories used to describe a person (or made available to a person to describe herself) are not obviously oppressive, repugnant, or prejudiced. They are untrue through inadequacy rather than inaccuracy: they do not "speak to the condition" of that person. She has experiences and perceptions, undergoes events, has to make choices or solve problems that are simply *not there* in the dominant narratives. She has to laboriously make these up for herself, if she can.

For this reason I prefer to include these, together with true counterstories, under the inclusive heading of reconstructive narratives. The first step in creating a reconstructive narrative, then, is to identify those bits of the master narrative that are false, misleading, overgeneralized, or entirely absent. The second is to retell the story in a way that recovers the features that the prevailing narrative denies, and that show people as moral agents worthy of respect. In the cases of master narratives that are directly oppressive, these recovered features show the marginalized lives as worthy of respect and self-respect. The master narrative of disabled mothers in which they are vulnerable, irresponsible, dependent on the state, and likely to end up exploiting their children as carers, can be retold in ways that remain true to the many additional problems a disabled woman may encounter in mothering, while also offering a tale in which she is thoughtful, ingenious, and protective of her kids. But in addition to countering the existing harmful narrative, there is also a narrative thread here that is *missing*. A reconstructive narrative might contribute the story line in which a disabled woman creatively assembles a collective of friends and supporters to supply the distinctive kinds of relationships she needs to function as a mother: her own equivalents of the socially recognized supports that make any parenting possible and for which numerous "parenting" stories are at hand.

Reconstructive narratives must be purposefully put together, perhaps not purely consciously or self-consciously, but in response to the wrongness or lack of the existing narrative. On occasion, wrongness may be noticed by an outsider who spots the discrepancy between expectation and experience, or the damage to identity and moral agency caused by it. But since in general people are skilled at ignoring and forgetting empirical information that conflicts with their beliefs,[1] it is more likely that a poor fit will be felt by the individual as the subjectively experienced wrongness of their lives running up against a toxic narrative, or foundering in the absence of one. However, reconstructive narratives aim not merely to reflect the truth of an individual's own experience (although that is useful in itself), but more generally to open up ontological possibilities for others as well. This means that although a reconstructive narrative will by definition be discordant with social norms, it still needs to have credibility within the group and outside it; it has to have some kind of empirical basis, and it must have psychological plausibility too.

THE MASTER NARRATIVES OF DISABILITY

Like other organizing categories such as gender or age, disability has a cluster of master narratives associated with it. These narratives prescribe individuals' behaviors, values, and life trajectories. As is generally the case for master narratives, the sources of the disability identities in common circulation are hard to discern. For one thing, they evolve: narratives in circulation are the mutant offspring of previous versions. Although one obvious place to find narratives is in the storytelling art forms of literature and drama, it is not that master narratives originate in books and films, but that they provide idealized and tidier versions of the identity narratives that circulate in society: this is why the literary versions make sense to us at all.

The themes of illness and impairment are not absent from fiction. Analyses of disability in literature look back to the stories of blind Tiresias and clubfooted Oedipus of mythology, and onward by way of Shakespeare's Richard III to more familiar nineteenth- and twentieth-century examples, like Captains Hook and Ahab. A number of authors in disability literary studies have identified distinct impairment narratives that appear in literature, cinema, and theater. Among the most prominent associated identities are the tragic victim; the hero overcoming the odds (the supercrip); the saintly sage; the sweet angel; the comic; the contaminant; the burden to society and family; and the evil or obsessive avenger, psychologically or morally warped by impairment (Norden 1995).[2] But there are very few *fictional* resources about disability that provide a good reconstructive narrative, a disability identity that is not damaging or limiting in the ways I have described. Crucially, these narratives are not often generated by disabled people themselves. They tell nondisabled people what they want to know, or think they want to know, about impairment. Because they satisfy the sense-making needs of nondisabled people, they are typically unconcerned with the brute realities of managing disability. In a review of the feature film *Passion Fish*, which depicts a paralyzed woman, André Dubus notes caustically that in "one scene in Louisiana, they're on a wharf and there's this little skiff, and she tells the nurse, 'Get me on the boat.' Next scene, she's in the boat, and I said, How the fuck did she lower this woman from the chair into the boat on the water? Show me that and you've got some story" (Smolens 1996, 5). In her memoir of disability activism, which I discuss in more detail in a moment, Simi Linton (2005) underscores how troubling nondisabled people find physical anomaly, and how strong is their drive to slot the impairment experience into a familiar frame of meaning. She describes being "faced with intrusive inquiries from strangers that began, 'what happened to you?' . . . with only the bits of information I give [the questioner] will nod and commiserate and act as if he now knows what is important to know about disability—its genesis" (Linton 2005, 110). Master narratives of disability, created in the main by nondisabled people, persist because of the comfort that they offer—they contain the anxiety that nondisabled, and often disabled people too, have about disability (Reeve 2002).

The primary harm of a toxic or missing narrative of disability identity is cultural, rather than economic or political. By "primary harm" I don't necessarily mean the most obvious harm. The economic, professional, and educational impact of impairment on people's lives is more easily spotted and quantified than the deleterious effects of attitudes. Nor are cultural harms necessarily the worst. Economic, educational, and vocational harms are real and significant and need to be addressed as issues of justice. Nevertheless, a psychoanalytic perspective on the dynamic between normality and impairment suggests that impairment, and especially the fear of one's own impairment, creates a level of

anxiety that must be defended against by a range of powerful, mostly unconscious mechanisms (Marks 1999). Although marginalization and outright oppression are obvious consequences of excluding disabled people, and in some
cases their carers (Kittay 1999), from social participation, I would argue that
disabling barriers don't spring up out of nowhere. They may appear in response to socioeconomic forces but they are held in place, sometimes for far
longer than is rational, by prevailing beliefs about the meaning of impairment.
These beliefs are culturally "carried" in the form of a repertoire of figurations
and stories about disabled people.

DISABILITY LITERATURE

Although crudely inspirational stories seem to have fallen out of favor in
the world of disability fiction, the baton has been taken up by real-life
memoirs (of which more in a moment). In fiction and film, what remains
are works in which the impairment is not central to the story; sometimes it
is there to make the character a bit more interesting (Hafferty and Foster
[1994] examine the deaf detectives in literature, for example), or it may be
used symbolically to reinforce the writer's theme (e.g., T. C. Boyles's *Talk
Talk*, 2006). There is another emerging genre in which the weirdness of
everyday life is conveyed through the perspective of narrators whose impairments give them a novel eye on the quotidian. A prime example here is
Mark Haddon's story of autism, *The Curious Incident of the Dog in the Night-
Time* (2003).

But the fictionalization of disability raises tricky epistemological questions
of voice and authority. Most fictional accounts are not written from direct personal experience. It is true that any writer of fiction draws on aspects of her experience to assemble characters and plots, and some writers will therefore be
able to refer to an impairment of their own, or to the knowledge acquired by
growing up with a disabled parent or sibling, or having a disabled child, or
even a disabled friend. These are all important perspectives on the phenomenon we call "disability," and they provide valid insights to complete the picture. However, their epistemological status cannot be the same as that of a person with subjective experience of life with an impairment. Lindemann Nelson
argues that good counterstories can be created either by or on behalf of the person whose identity is in need of this kind of work. Rarely, an outsider is better
placed to offer a reconstructive narrative, so that a person who has lived in a
country that offers wider opportunities to mobility-impaired people may be
able to give an account of possible lives that could not be imagined by wheelchair users elsewhere. Nevertheless, the appropriation of a socially marginalized group's experience for literary purposes must raise disquiet. In general,
marginalized groups have lacked control over their own representation, and

their "long history of multiple, cross-cutting systems of domination and sub-ordination" means that members of marginalized groups cannot and maybe should not trust other people to supply good imagery or narrative (Meyers 1994, 103) that subvert ingrained stereotypes.

The use of disability in fiction intended for a nondisabled audience also raises the question of how much reader recognition compromises truthful reporting. Assuming that most readers' ideas about disability derive from socially circulating master narratives, readers will expect and even need to see those threads in the story in order to recognize it for what it is. For the author not to baffle her audience, she will have to draw from those famil-iar narratives to some extent, even if her eventual aim is to challenge or re-sist them. By contrast, the author who identifies herself as disabled authen-ticates what might be an unfamiliar representation with the epistemic authority of her own life.[3]

To say that it is illegitimate for a nondisabled author to write about im-pairment would be to confuse the aim of fiction with the aims of politics or psychotherapy. A writer generally has interests other than transforming so-cial or personal realities. As I discussed in chapter 3, the practice of making moral judgments frequently demands the conscious extension beyond per-sonal experience, an imaginative projection into another's lifeworld. Good fictional accounts of disability have often served to extend the boundaries of moral empathy for nondisabled readers. Poor fictional accounts, however, have just as often reinforced stereotypes and foreclosed moral imagination. And even good fiction is less likely to provide radical resistance to prevailing toxic stories, or offer a narrative that is missing, or describe the practical as-pects of managing everyday life with an impairment.

DISABILITY MEMOIRS

We are in ethically much less troublesome territory with the disability memoir. Unlike fiction, autobiographical accounts necessarily have episte-mological authority, even if the account does not claim to be representative of everyone, everywhere, with a specific impairment. One exception here is the account written by the parent of a disabled child (less commonly, the partner of a disabled adult). These raise similar unease about control and voice as fiction does. These accounts (for example, Paul West on his deaf daughter [1969], Bérubé on his son with Down syndrome [1996], and Dan Kennedy on his daughter with restricted growth [2003]) are firsthand ac-counts of parenting a child with an impairment, not of the experience of the impairment itself. It is crucial to keep this distinction in mind. As I have indicated, I consider the parental account to be one we need to have, but it is not the same as that of the child or adult. The problem here is that very

often the parental account is the *only* one we have: where there is severe intellectual impairment, or the child dies, the disabled person is not in any
position to provide a complementary story. Disability memoir here reflects
the real-life tensions that exist in the disability world between disabled people who are well able to articulate their desires and demands, given the
chance, and parents of disabled children or adults who, because of their age
or impairment, cannot.

The fiction of disability has been overtaken by a recent upsurge in impairment memoirs, a subset of the widely popular suffering/confessional
genre that includes accounts of cancer and other diseases (Fox, *Lucky Man*),
mental illness (Keyser, *Girl, Interrupted*), self-harm (Leatham, *Bloodletting*),
eating disorders (Hornbacher, *Wasted*), or addictions (Wurtzel, *More, Now,
Again*; Zailckas, *Smashed*). Still, the bulk of this literature is about illness,
and although it is not always possible to differentiate illness and disability,
there remain major and morally significant differences between them. In
his groundbreaking analysis of illness narratives, *The Wounded Storyteller*
(1995), Arthur Frank described serious illness as "a loss of the 'destination
and map' that had previously grounded the ill person's life," which is also
apposite for a person becoming impaired in adolescence or adulthood after a certain stability of identity has been achieved. For Frank, "the illness
story begins in wreckage," and his analysis then deals with how this "wreckage" is restored through being "transformed into *another kind* of narrative."
In these transitional situations, says Frank, ill or abruptly disabled people
"have to learn to 'think differently.'" It is important that he says *think* rather
than *behave* or *manage*, because alongside practical behavioral change, the
restoration demands cognitive and affective work too. His typology identifies three categories of illness narrative: restitution stories, in which the
present incapacity is a blip in an otherwise normal life course; chaos narratives, in which all structure is lost and which, says Frank, can only really be
described in hindsight after some kind of order is restored; and quest narratives, where illness catalyzes a journey of self-discovery. Quest narratives
are then subdivided into the memoir (illness story combined with the facts
of a life), the manifesto (closer to a political account), and automythology
(where the author undergoes such massive disruption that she "not only
has survived but has been reborn") (123).

Now some kinds of disability story readily fit into Frank's typology. Accounts of the writer's impairment by a stroke or car accident, followed by
successful reentry into a (different kind of) life, would count as automythology, with—as we shall see—in some cases a substantial touch of
manifesto. Where Frank's scheme proves inadequate is that illness is first
encountered as a *disruption* of an already established normality. Even if illness persists so that eventually it becomes the person's new normality, there
remains a prior life to look back on and with which to compare a present

state. To a reader, the piquancy of the account lies mostly in the contrast between life before and life after the onset of illness. But where do we place the experience of *always having been* different? Being propelled by illness or accident out of one's accustomed state of being into an unknown and unwanted one, with all the associated losses and accommodations, is a very different experience from growing up with the awareness that one's normality is, in the eyes of the mainstream world, abnormal. The experiences of late-onset conditions like Huntington's disease or slowly progressive disorders like cystic fibrosis are different again.

A look at the published memoirs suggests there are two biases. First, a disproportionality in number: there are far more illness than disability narratives. Thomas Couser makes the perceptive point that illness is easier for "normal" readers to identify with, not just because it is more familiar, but because it is easier psychically in that the illness narrative is often a story of restitution. The existential threat to the reader is distanced because restitution ensures a happy ending. But because disabilities are ongoing (there is generally no recovery), it is harder to "find a vantage point for narrative, a safe distance from an ongoing and sometimes consuming condition" (Couser 1997, 183). Second, the range of published disability experiences is dismayingly limited.[4] So many are about the experience of posttraumatic paraplegia or quadriplegia that "paralysis bids to become the paradigmatic form of physical disability," probably because "its obviousness, extremity, and apparent intractability . . . so dramatically threaten one's sense of integrity and may so radically rupture one's sense of autobiographical continuity" (184). These narratives are examples of automythology: an interruption of one identity and its restoration or reconstitution.

By contrast, what I call "steady state disability stories," about conditions that are present from birth or childhood and change relatively little, fail to fit the conventional story arc of crisis and resolution. This may partly account for their scarcity: to be a good story, something needs to go awry. When we are schooled in a narrative tradition of opposition, struggle, and triumph, it is hard to recognize an account of a life lived differently, with no distinct crisis and no major change other than getting older, as being a story worth listening to. For their part the authors of this experience, for whom it is their normality, may feel less driven to make sense of it or to articulate it to others through writing. Authors of "steady state" or "unexciting slow decline" memoirs have to get around this somehow. As we shall see in a moment, one way is to turn it from a story of physical crisis and recovery into an account of emerging political self-consciousness and radicalization.

The disability memoir genre is not vast, but still large enough for a proper overview to warrant more space than I can give here. Instead, I will use representative memoirs to illustrate some of the features they share, and others where there is less commonality.

Life Interrupted

Simi Linton is a psychologist and activist whose autobiographical *My Body Politic* describes her life after she became paraplegic in a car accident in 1971. She begins the book with a retelling of the accident itself, which also killed her best friend and her husband. Immediately afterward she spent some time in a rehabilitation center, then studied for a while in New York, before moving to Berkeley and becoming involved in the work of the Center for Independent Living there. Linton's book therefore follows a conventional narrative structure, beginning with the "wreck" separating predisabled from disabled identities, and then charting her physical restoration of health and her reentry to the world, and culminating in a kind of second rebirth, this time into political consciousness. In Frank's typology it is an example of automythology.

By contrast, John Hockenberry's *Moving Violations* starts at what might be taken as the point of his maximal postdisablement normalization: when as a reporter for National Public Radio he covered the Kurdish refugee exodus in 1991. Unlike Linton again, Hockenberry presents himself as a classic supercrip, investing (it seems) huge physical and psychic effort in doing anything that a nonparaplegic man could do, and doing it at least as well and preferably much better. His difference from Linton is exemplified in their reactions to the Berkeley Center for Independent Living. Where she seems to have found liberation and a welcoming community, Hockenberry writes that, when deciding which university to apply to, "I had heard that Berkeley, California was a mecca for the disabled [but] in my view, any school that would go out of its way to attract crips must have something wrong with it, so I immediately ruled out Berkeley" (Hockenberry 1995, 115). Hockenberry is more self-avowedly independent, less inclined to identify with the mass of disability, and at least initially, his professional success entailed hiding the fact of his impairment from his employers. Linton was politically involved in the anti-war movement before her accident, and she is convinced that it was by joining with disabled people in activism that she acquired what she needed in her new life. Again unlike Hockenberry, she acknowledges periods of depression, loneliness, and failure in her postaccident life.

Yet despite these and other differences, the two accounts have a lot in common. Interestingly, the features they share are often those points that do not appear in nondisabled writing about traumatic disablement. Both accounts embrace a broadly social model of disability and both recognize the connection between disability and other forms of social exclusion: of black people (in Hockenberry) or of women and sexual minorities (in Linton). They manage scrupulously to identify the social and cultural barriers against disabled people while not losing sight of the impairment and impairment effects on the individual and others around them. Both authors are at pains to show how their experience paradoxically combined both abrupt disjunction between the former life and the new one, with a lengthy process of learning how to *be* the new identity. Hockenberry describes this as "the quantum view of disability [that] allows you to dare to think that you can have lived two lives, two bodies occupying two places at once. Suddenly, in an instant, radical change: I was different, yet I was still the same person" (Hockenberry 1995, 26). Linton tells us that although "[t]he new shape and formation of my body were set on that April day," her life as a disabled person is one she grew into: "The meaning this new body would have for me took years to know" (Linton 2005, 3).

Hockenberry especially stresses the labor that goes into becoming and being disabled, "the hard work and painstaking efforts taken over the past 19 years to relearn a physical life" (Hockenberry 1995, 27). There is nothing passive about this transition. It is a struggle, and in the process bodily normativity is radically altered. Discovering that habitual actions were no longer possible meant working out an alternative: "You could imagine the tragedy of never being able to do things, only to discover there was a way to do them after all" (30). It is not just the relearning of everyday activities (how do I get up steps?), but a theoretical restructuring as well: "Finding a personal concept of normal in a place where nurses patrolled your urethra was the main task in the hospital. . . . The concept of what is normal became quite foggy and obscure" (30). It's from Hockenberry too that we get a clear sense of the intellectual challenge that comes with being differently embodied: "Far from being a blank wall of misery, my body now presented an intriguing puzzle of great depth and texture. To rediscover my changed body was to explore the idea of a body and its relationship to the mind in a way that no night class, self-help book, or therapist could." Similarly, Linton describes the intense engagement with the reality of the body's parameters that went into acquiring the new way of being: "I had gotten to this place not by denying my disability or, implausibly, 'overcoming' it, but by sailing headlong into it. Making sense of it had become the most meaningful thing I could do" (Linton 2005, 120).

Both authors stress the inadequacy of information available from official sources. Linton and the others at her rehabilitation center were faced not just with a new situation but with a way of being that was radically unfamiliar: "None of us knew anyone else like us out there. Even at the hospital only a handful of the people we saw working there had disabilities. . . . Were we 'handicapped'? What was that? What would it mean for us? What would we call ourselves?" (18). Other disabled people were the carriers of this knowledge: "There was another curriculum we needed access to—we needed the tools and knowledge that experienced disabled people have. We were novices" (109); "in my early years with disability, I was flying by the seat of my pants, and so many say they did the same" (159). They acquired their survival information from each other, particularly for difficult or taboo subjects: "Most of us had sustained spinal cord injuries to our necks or backs, others had brain injuries. All of us were radically altered in the way we moved, felt our bodies, responded to sexual stimulation. . . . This group of relative strangers, women and men, adolescents, married people, probably both gay and straight people (though no one said that they were gay), we shared our stories . . . so when questions about sex came up, we turned to each other. 'What did you hear?' 'Can we get any books?' 'What happened when you went home last weekend?' We could start putting the pieces together" (11–12).

They needed the tools and knowledge of other disabled people because the outsider knowledge, even of professionals like the medical staff, was useless. Important points were absent or presented in unintelligible ways. Usable strategies for survival were not available through the common stock of whole or part narratives. Hockenberry is particularly scathing about the standard narratives open to disabled people, and the rigid parameters that determine what nondisabled readers and viewers are to be told. "There are endless role model profiles of famous heroic quadriplegic skiers and football players. . . . The hero business is targeted largely at the nondisabled. It's apparently reassuring to be told over and over again that you can survive a disabling injury and live off the sale of the TV movie. But what about practical details from people who know the ropes, who have hung in there, who have taken the airline flights, gotten a real job, and found the unfindable public bathroom?" (Hockenberry 1995, 137). Both Hockenberry and Linton are clear that, within the bigger existential narrative, the banalities of toileting, tiredness, and sex are key to constructing a flourishing identity as a disabled person.

These memoirs count as reconstructive because although set within a familiar narrative structure of crisis and resolution—the car crash, paraplegia, and eventual rehabilitation into the world outside the hospital—the stories are played out with unexpected insights into detail and into their wider context. In this way they consciously challenge and subvert inaccurate, and therefore morally unhelpful, narratives of disability, by offering an account that is more shaded and ambiguous. So the conventional postaccident normative staging of shock, denial, grief, and mourning is conspicuous by its absence. There *is* shock and despair, but they seem outweighed by curiosity and attention to the work of reembodiment. Neither Linton nor Hockenberry seems to have spent much time raging against fate or denying what had happened. Linton is clear that this is a mixed blessing: "I sometimes felt sad not to walk or run or dance, but I didn't argue with it, or bemoan my fate, or desperately look for cures. My frenzy, it seemed, was about making it on the road I was on . . . there was denial mixed in all this, I can see that now, but there was also acceptance" (Linton 2005, 31–32).

Both Hockenberry and Linton know that what they are doing is rewriting a tragedy/triumph story with different claims about what counts as tragedy and as triumph, versions that are closer to their own, less neatly packaged experience. The reconstruction of counterstory and new narrative are in Linton's growing politicization, Hockenberry's moments of identification with marginalized blacks, the rejection of the standard tropes of either denying or "overcoming," the insistence on giving precise details about how access to buildings or employment is barred, and the insistence that their disablement entails both losses and gains: both of them acknowledge the role disability played in giving them professional drive and focus, and in Linton's case a community of other disabled people.

Steady State and Slow Decline

Harriet McBryde Johnson's *Too Late to Die Young* also counts as a reconstructive narrative. Unlike Linton's and Hockenberry's accounts, it lacks the structure of crisis and transition, and so exemplifies the difficulty of writing about the experience of impairment when that experience is part of the writer's normality. Johnson's condition (which she nowhere identifies by name) is present from birth, and although her physical state has deteriorated over time, there is no trajectory of disruption/reconstitution. She trained as a lawyer and gradually became involved in disability law, so that instead of changes in her physical condition, the book tracks changes in her stance toward her own impairment, and political changes that Johnson (and others) has brought about. As a result, her book is more accessible to nondisabled readers and probably more likely to offer an alternative narrative of identity to them than to disabled people. It functions less as a practical how-to-manage-this guide than Linton's and Hockenberry's, and more as a template for what Johnson believes to be a form of life morally worth living for a disabled person. A good part of the *resistance* in the narrative offered by Johnson, however, lies in her counterintuitive staking of a claim to enjoyment in impairment: "When nondisabled people start learning about disability, what seems most startling, most difficult to accept, is the possibility of pleasure. . . . We need to confront the life-killing stereotype that says we're all about suffering. We need to bear witness to our pleasures. I'm talking in part about the pleasures we share with nondisabled people [where there is] no impairment: disability makes no difference. But I'm also talking about those pleasures that are peculiarly our own, that are so bound up with our disabilities that we wouldn't experience them, or wouldn't experience them the same way, without our disabilities" (Johnson 2006, 253–54).

Henry Kisor has been hearing impaired from birth and his autobiography, *What's That Pig Outdoors?* (1990), is the story of his career in journalism. Like Johnson, and unlike Linton and Hockenberry, Kisor lacks a "before" against which to compare an "after." In his account, hearing
impairment is not displayed through a contrast with hearing people, but in
the practices that Kisor has to invent in order to manage education, work,
and private life when all of these are organized around the presumption of
hearing. Kisor's job means his deafness becomes problematic in certain circumstances; although writing does not require the ability to hear, other aspects of journalism, like interviewing or making arrangements by telephone
before the era of e-mail, do. And in these rather particular circumstances,
Kisor details his strategies for survival as a deaf journalist in a mostly hearing world. The most prominent thing in this part of Kisor's story is, again,
the time and effort it takes to work up these strategies and his sense that he
is doing so in isolation. Because he was born into a hearing family, his identity is not as a Deaf person but as a "regular guy" who can't hear, and like
Hockenberry, he tries for as long as he can to "pass."

So although Kisor's book overtly offers a very positive narrative for deaf
people, its implicit moral lesson is how important it is not to be, or be seen
to be, different from a hearing person. The phenomenon of "passing" has
been extensively examined in the context of the other social marginalities
of ethnicity, sexual orientation, and gender identity. Marginal and excluded
people pass "when they take up the [dominant] group's norms for themselves, even though they don't 'really' conform to those norms" (Lindemann Nelson 2001, 126). One prerequisite for passing to be at all possible
is that the person must look or behave closely enough to the norm to be
taken for it, albeit with some effort and subterfuge, as in the case of the
light-skinned mixed-race woman's efforts to claim a southern European an-
cestry, or the gay man marrying in order to be taken for straight. People with
various kinds of impairment also try, more or less willingly, to ensure that
their bodily form and function match the social norm. "Function" here
means both straightforward physical acts—walking, picking objects up—
and social functions such as being able to work an eight-hour day, communicate with others in certain ways, and so on. The demands of "passing"
are stringent: the accommodations are all on the side of the disabled person, they must be not or only minimally apparent to other people, and they
must not disturb conventional social arrangements. The aim is to be taken
for normal. Internalized by the disabled person, this becomes the demand
that nothing about one's impairment should "show." Some impairments
are not visible, and depending on circumstances, even severe physical impairment can sometimes be hidden from view. The rise of e-mail and text
messaging has enabled many hearing-impaired people not only to communicate easily with each other, but to communicate with hearing people

on a much more equal basis than before. Their hearing impairment becomes something under their control to disclose, to choose whether to make it part of their self-presentation to others. Similarly, John Hockenberry could pass to his first employers because, as he was a radio station journalist, they never saw him. They were unaware of his mobility impairment until the day he missed a deadline because he could not find an accessible public telephone (this was in olden times before mobile phones, children). If it is really impossible to hide the impairment altogether, as it is for many impairments, then the aim of passing is to manage it so that others can forget it, at least temporarily.

Now one line of argument says there is nothing wrong about the desire to pass. We all want to be valued by others for things like the skills we bring to a job or the personal characteristics we bring to a friendship. We'd want those features to be predominant in our interactions, so that people leave the meeting thinking, "She chairs the committee so well," not, "She's so blind, and still she chairs this committee well." Yet the urge to pass often goes beyond a reasonable desire for respect and autonomy of self-presentation, and into altogether murkier territory about shame and fear. Can an identity in which passing plays a major role be morally laudable? Can an identity *narrative* in which passing plays a major role be morally exemplary? What does it do to moral agency, or society's capacity to recognize alternative forms of agency? These questions—which I am not going to take on here—raise some doubts about the kind of identity narrative Kisor's memoir provides.

In contrast is an account that highlights as much as possible the anomaly of its author's mode of "hearing." Michael Chorost has been hearing impaired from early childhood, so one layer of his narrative is about always being different, but on top of that it is a transition paralleling those of Linton and Hockenberry. When he is thirty-six, his hearing impairment abruptly and unexpectedly increases, to the extent that he is unable to function as he had in his previous normality (which, we note, was an abnormal state in conventional terms). He opts to have a cochlear implant. Because of his perceptiveness and literary skill, Chorost's account is enormously informative both to hearing people with no knowledge of deafness, and to any hearing-impaired person curious about cochlear implants. Of all the memoirs discussed here, Chorost's is by far the most self-analytical about identity. He examines the physical and psychological processes he underwent in becoming a cochlear implant user. Early on he asks himself rhetorically how he will get "through the change." For his answer he instinctively turns to narrative: "As a lifelong reader of literature, I already had some answers to hand. A mind richly stocked with stories can select from them as needed, applying narrative to the chaos of experience in order to move ahead with greater sureness to an imagined resolution. . . . I needed a story not of survival, but of transformation" (Chorost 2005, 26).

Some reviews of the book described it as a story of the transition from hearing impairment to hearing, and indeed the subtitle of the paperback version is *My Journey Back to the Hearing World*. And yet Chorost explicitly says that this is not what the implantation was about. Rather it is about acquiring and learning how to use a novel way of processing auditory input. This is neither a narrative of restoration nor of passing. In fact, his transformation, although one that comes about by choice, is as disruptive to his former normality as spinal cord lesion was for Hockenberry and Linton. Far from being restored to the hearing world, or even to his prior hearing impairment, he considers that he has become something new: "I had most definitely not reacquired my *self*" (Chorost 2005, 83).

Like Kisor and Hockenberry, and unlike Linton and Johnson, Chorost is a lone wolf. His book is about addressing a problem somatically located in an individual's ears. The sole form of collective identity that either Kisor or Chorost refers to is the signing Deaf community, Kisor with a guarded politeness, Chorost with a kind of wistfulness; but both are outside it, and neither shows a desire to incorporate either the Deaf or the disabled communities into their own identities. The collective is not the subject of their stories.

Earlier, I suggested that reconstructive narratives can offer (1) alternative and morally less harmful accounts, (2) information or strategies that disabled people need to survive and flourish that are missing from existing accounts, and (3) accounts that are entirely missing from the existing repertoire. By these criteria the memoirs I discuss have varying degrees of success. The three that involve reconstitution of a prior identity do not challenge the conventional reading of events (interruption and remaking of a life), but they do give an alternative version of what reconstitution entails. The picture of a passive process of recovery assisted by wheelchairs or cochlear implants, for instance, is replaced by a portrayal of the active engagement of body and will; curiosity and tenacity replace resignation and patience as core virtues. The narrative reconstructions by Linton, Hockenberry, and Chorost, through the "attention to particularity" (Somers 1994, 634) inherent in narrative identity, call our attention to forms of agency that, because they fail to fit normative patterns, otherwise go unrecognized.

Kisor offers an alternative identity of a professionally successful deaf man, and his account also contains practical strategies to help others learn how to follow his example. But his uncritical acceptance of the need to pass in the hearing world means that although his account has virtues as a counterstory and offers some practical information on how to get by, it cannot count as a transformative one. Both Chorost and Johnson are more radical in that they provide *new* narrative identities that were previously lacking in the repertoire. In Chorost's case this is largely because the technology is too new for enough narratives of cochlear implantation to have been written. Johnson's radicalness lies not just in her political engagement but in what appears to have been a lifelong self-assured refusal to accept others' representations of herself and her body, and in her celebration of the possibility of enjoying phenotypic variation, even one as extreme as hers.

ETHICAL IMPLICATIONS

Morally preferable identity narratives are those that enhance the moral agency of the people they involve. This is a basic ethical criterion (although not the only one: another is that enhancing the moral agency of one marginalized group should not decrease another's).[5] In order to enhance moral agency effectively, the story must be as phenomenologically or empirically faithful as possible to people's experiences. Accurate experiential accounts like these contribute to the cultural database of identity narratives about the lives of people with impairment. The end ethical goal is that they should displace more damaging portrayals and insert ones that are missing. The argument is sometimes made that a more powerful way to counter the wrong of toxic identity stories is to *overcorrect* with a stronger version that is not necessarily empirically accurate, in other words, to make idealized claims, downplaying the effect of impairment on a disabled person's quality of life, or exaggerating the political unanimity of the disability community. However, although these idealized versions might be effective in the short term and useful in defined applications (as part of a political campaign, for instance), in the longer term they are less likely to transform the sociocultural set of stories about how people with impairments can really flourish in our society. Over time, as the discrepancy between the idealized version and empirical reality is noticed, the idealized versions will lose credibility among nondisabled people, and they will fail to mesh with the experienced reality of impairment. Disabled people whose lives do not match the ideal script—who are not supercrips or perpetually feisty disabled activists—will be damaged by this failure too. The idealized counterstory will rapidly become as harmful as any of the "bad" narratives it was designed to replace.

But a theory of narrative identity will also run into trouble if it considers that a narrative (and an identity associated with it) must always be consistent or unified. Some writers on identity hold that the function of narrative is to pull together an otherwise impossibly incoherent set of perceptions and experiences, so that the self's unity (which they take as a prerequisite for selfhood) "resides in the unity of a narrative" (MacIntyre 1985, 205). Indeed, Diana Tietjens Meyers argues that in their self narratives, people can weave together the otherwise incompatible facets highlighted by different models of the self: the rational, Kantian, unitary, or communitarian self, the permanently conflicted self of psychoanalysis, the feminist relational self, or the embodied self (Meyers 2004). Arthur Frank suggests something similar when he

argues that chaos narratives are in fact *unnarratable* because chaos, by definition, cannot be contained within an orderly structure. But the reasoning that
a narrative identity must imply adherence to a single story that is coherent
and complete in itself is false. Lives are always more fragmented and partially
chaotic than this. A narrative of identity may be broken by events requiring
the reconstitution of a new identity, as we have seen in Linton's and Hockenberry's writing, or a subjectivity may be best expressed through a thread of
multiple narratives running parallel, crossing, and fading in and out of significance over time, as in Johnson's. To deny this is to risk "denying all those
aspects of the self that contradict the ideal of unity" (Alford 1991, 188). Although Alford seems to think constructing an artificially unified account is acceptable if done "in full awareness that it is partial, provisional, serving to give
the illusion of unity to what is actually a fragmented subject" (187), the question is whether most of us genuinely are or can be "in full awareness" when
we do this. However accurate and morally good the story, then, we may still
be doing something epistemically and ethically wrong by splitting off or
denying perceptions or forms of experience that are incompatible with an idealized story, or not containable within the conventional ordering of a narrative. Drawing on modernist and postrealist fiction, Maureen Whitebrook has
argued that less conventional forms of narrative have the ability to cope with
disorder and fragmentation. In terms of identity, then, coherence "does not
necessarily equate to unbroken narrative flow" (Whitebrook 2001, 119). Narrative identity indeed may be more tolerant of indeterminacy, disjunction,
and ongoing reinterpretation—all of which can figure prominently in the experiences of disabled people—than we generally assume.

    If moral identity is created in part through narrative, then which stories
are available, and to whom, becomes a matter of ethical responsibility. Collectively, our ethical responsibility is to keep the fullest possible range of
nontoxic narratives of identity in circulation, in accessible forms, and to ensure that toxic ones are identified, and countered or replaced, wherever they
arise. For the individual, once we become conscious of the uses of narrative,
then a new form of moral agency—the astute choice of the right narrative—
becomes possible. With it, a new personal moral responsibility seems to be
laid upon us: to choose, as far as choice comes into it, the narrative that best
tells the truth of one's life.

    Now Arthur Frank suggests that telling the truth of one's life is an ethical
imperative, not simply for the sake of one's own self-determination and
moral agency, but for others: "Storytelling is *for* an other just as much as it
is for oneself" (1995, 17). But before we get too carried away here, we need
to recall that for many disabled people (globally, probably *most* disabled
people) this is an impossibly tough order. The world over, disabled people
face enough of a struggle to live reasonably well in the face of social exclusion, limited education or employment, poverty, and in some cases fatigue,

pain, or depression; the last thing we need is to shoulder the responsibility for a social project of reconstructive self-narrative. In reality, of course, the individual ethical burden of choosing a morally wholesome identity stories is made considerably lighter by a realistic appraisal of the possibilities of self-narration. The freedom to make yourself up as you wish is severely constrained by other internal and cultural forces, some of which were discussed earlier. As Lindemann Nelson says, storytelling, however powerful, is not the only thing.

To talk of identity as narratively constituted immediately implies the need for both narrator and listener(s). To whom the story is being told, and the aim of telling, have political implications. Narratives about disability identity of the kind we have looked at in this chapter offer an alternative framework around which the meaning of impairment can take shape in individuals' lives, but many in the disability movement and social movement theory now suggest that they also offer "a basis for identity politics, allowing people with different disabilities to tell a story about their common cause" (Siebers 2005, 8). The following chapter takes a look at the ethical pros and cons of a political disability identity.

NOTES

1. The psychological literature on this is extensive. Overviews of memory and forgetting may be found in Schachter (2001).

2. For more on disability in literature, theater, and film, see Kriegel (1987); Eberly (1988); Cumberbatch and Negrine (1992); Hevey (1992); Norden (1995); Ross (1997); Darke (1998); and Stemp (2004).

3. Note that this is not a claim that personal experience gives absolute authority to an account; merely that knowing it is "really true" will tend to reassure the reader when she encounters something unsettling.

4. The same can be said of illness narratives. A look at any illness bibliography shows a heavy bias toward stories of cancer recovery.

5. However, a proportionate reduction in the freedom of operation of the dominant group would in principle be acceptable. This requires a fuller discussion of justice and social policy than I am able to go into here.

7

Political Recognition and Misrecognition

> We are all bound together, not by this list of our collective symptoms but by the social and political circumstances that have forged us as a group.
>
> —Simi Linton

> To portray a group is to engage in a political activity.
>
> —Harlan Lane

In this book I have been asking questions about the embodied experience of impairment and its effect on disabled people's moral subjectivity. The previous chapter used examples from disability memoirs to consider how the private identities of individual disabled people are formed, in part, by selecting from among the culturally available narratives about disability. In addition to having commonalities at the individual level, however, the authors of the memoirs I looked at vary markedly in their attention to the *collective* dimension of impairment. Where Hockenberry, Kisor, and Chorost tell their stories from the perspective of themselves as individuals, the narratives of Linton and Johnson interweave their personal biographies with an intense consciousness of and growing commitment to disabled people in general, and to what some people call the disability community.

This chapter reflects on the ethical consequences of a collective disability identity. Many bioethicists will consider this a question of politics more than ethics and argue that it does not fall within bioethics' remit. In counterargument I suggest first that the existence (or not) of a disability community has significance for the identities of disabled people and therefore for their moral and political agency as well. Second, the recognition of a collective disability identity by nondisabled people has practical and epistemological effects on the ability of disabled people to articulate their desires and needs. Third, if a political collective identity proves to be a suitable vehicle for enhancing the agency of a traditionally disadvantaged group, there is an ethical requirement to support it. Disability studies has now produced a lot of work on the politicization of collective disability action, and alongside it stands a large body of insightful political philosophy theorizing group identities of different kinds. There is still a need for a thoroughgoing attempt to place disability as a political identity within those theoretical frameworks, but that is not what I want to do in this chapter. My aim here is more modest: to consider some of the ethical work that a collective disability identity can do. I will not be discussing the political function of minority group recognition in any detail, as my primary interest here is to explore the effect of collective identification as disabled on the moral understandings of disabled and nondisabled people.

COLLECTIVE IDENTITIES AND RECOGNITION

The concept of a collective disability identity needs to be distinguished from the identities, or in the terms of chapter 6, identity narratives, which individual disabled people develop. I've been contending that people incorporate their bodily experiences into their individual senses of self, identity, and subjectivity, and that variant embodied experience may contribute to disabled people having distinct moral perceptions. I make much more tentative claims for the role of collective identity, partly because the debates around it are so complex and contested, but also because even if there is such a thing, a "disability identity" has been around for too short a time for theorists to start making extensive claims about what it does.

One way of characterizing social groups is on the basis of how voluntary the association of its members is. What are called "found communities" are the groups and neighborhoods into which we are born and grow up (Friedman 1992). Communitarian ethicists tend to consider found communities, together with the family unit, as the primary ground of personal identity and moral understanding. Marilyn Friedman agrees with this as a picture of early moral life, but she also holds that for many people there comes a time when they choose to form different kinds of bonds, and enter other communities, in order to relocate and renegotiate the various constituents of their identities (Friedman 1992, 95). In the terminology of the previous chapter, they want to take up a different story about themselves.

An important ethical function of both found and chosen groups is their ability to articulate interests, needs, and desires that would otherwise be invisible or neglected. Marginalized and stigmatized groups embody and, under the right conditions, articulate ethical tensions within a society. It should be clear from earlier discussions that the embodiment of disabled perspectives is as significant here as their overt articulation. However, if we do want disabled people's perspectives expressed in a way that gets them on the political agenda with the aim of improving matters, then there need to be some kind of political consciousness and appropriate vehicles for expressing it.

Ethical analyses of identity politics focus primarily on how the political recognition of a minority group helps to rectify the long-standing injustices its members have suffered. Much of the most insightful work on the ethical function of recognizing marginal political identities comes from feminist and postcolonial theorists; in feminist political philosophy the work of Nancy Fraser and Iris Marion Young, and the often vigorous debate between them, has been particularly influential. Although disagreeing on many points, both Fraser and Young agree that *redistribution* and *recognition* make distinct contributions to social remediation (Fraser 2000; Young 2000). Redistribution of resources corrects economic injustice, which is by far the easier face of injustice to spot and the one to which disability activism has given most attention. But Fraser, Young, and others also acknowledge that justice for a disadvantaged group requires social and cultural recognition, and equally that transforming the cultural status of a group generally has consequences for its socioeconomic status as well. These authors see such sociocultural recognition essentially as a prerequisite for making the appropriate political responses to "structural inequalities that disadvantage" a group (Young 2000, 105). In *Justice and the Politics of Difference* (1990), Young argues that while economically and socially oppressive practices unfairly benefit some groups over others in material ways, they also foster the very patterns of belief that enable unjust social practices and institutions to be taken for granted. Indeed, it seems plausible that the beliefs come first developmentally, deriving much of their power and persistence from unconscious processes of defense and projection that have been identified as operating in the context of disability and other "others" (Marks 1999).

Scholars who favor the concept of recognition will argue that being recognized as a group with legitimate political claims is ethically desirable, not because it is necessarily ontologically true—that there really is a bunch of people out there who *are* that—but because having the concept at hand enables structural injustices to be corrected.[1] But for other theorists, among them Charles Taylor (1994) and Axel Honneth (1996), sociocultural recognition does much more than simply enable civic authorities to know to whom they should give the goods. These theorists take the view that persistent denigration, stigmatization, or refusal to admit the existence of a group are ethical wrongs because of the effects on the group's members. Because they believe that social recognition is crucial to the proper formation of the self, they consider that its refusal causes harm to the self's capacity for moral and political agency. This interpretation of identity politics accepts that "obstacles to the self-development of individuals, and to the formation and exercise of their agency, emerge in complex cultural and psychic forms, as well as through more familiar kinds of socio-economic inequality" (Kenny 2004, 40).

Not surprisingly perhaps, the idea that members of subordinated groups are subjected to moral harm as much through lack of acknowledgment as through being out of work or in poor housing has met some resistance. Critics object that moral subjectivities are not such tender plants, and to suggest that they are is to forget that "individuals forge a sense of themselves as much by rejecting and refining collective identity as by immersion in it" (Kenny 2004, 157). What this objection misses, though, is a point I made earlier: that the idea of self-identification with a community or group as a conscious choice is based on a modernist, liberal picture of the individual and her relationship to social structures. If that picture is inadequate then it becomes less certain that rejecting, refining, or immersing oneself in a collective identity can ever be performed as cleanly or as rationally as this. The point that I take Taylor and others to be making is that processes of identity formation are always multilayered, and many aspects of it are not open to conscious choice or manipulation. As a result, the real, damaging effects of nonrecognition are likely to remain obscured precisely because subjects do not "forge a sense of themselves" in a way that allows them knowingly to correct for gaps or distortions.

A more telling objection to the *social nonrecognition damages individual moral capacity* hypothesis comes from theorists who are unconvinced that a psychosocial model about individual subjectivity can be scaled up to apply to collective identities. Seyla Benhabib, for instance, finds it "both theoretically wrong and politically dangerous to conflate the individual's search for the expression of his/her unique identity with the politics of identity" (2002, 53). The two quests for identity and agency may, as we saw in the discussion of hearing-impaired children and the Deaf community, come into conflict. These critics would argue that while a disabled person's agency may be harmed by direct acts of discrimination or violence against her, or by being told that her understanding of her own life is wrong, she is not affected in the same way by stigmatization of disabled people in general. This objection seems a little too broad to be convincing. It is true that the domains of individual identity and political identity should not be equated with each other, and that elision from one to another occurs rather easily in academic literature and political rhetoric. But it seems less convincing that a general atmosphere of disrespect or hostility toward disabled people can really fail to touch the self-respect of a disabled person, even if she only observes disrespect shown toward other disabled people and never experiences it herself. A hearing-impaired person may never be faced with direct mockery, for instance, but will almost certainly have seen deaf people (especially old deaf people) being used for comic effect in films and television programs; it is reasonable to suppose that this causes harm to her self-image, albeit in different ways than harm caused directly to her person.

At the turn of the twenty-first century Nancy Fraser began to reject the conflation of recognition with identity politics (Fraser 2000), fearing that it produces too great a concentration on getting the identity "right" before embarking on the redistribution of resources, effectively distracting from efforts at redistribution while at the same time creating pressure to reify group identities that are not really up to bearing that weight. Rather than looking to group-specific identity, then, she links recognition to what she calls the "social status," by which she means the ability of group members to participate equally in social life. For those who are disturbed by the psychic or cultural biases of the politics of recognition, this reconfiguration has the advantage that harm is not "relayed through free-floating cultural representations or discourses" but through social institutions that regard "some categories of social actors as normative and others as deficient or inferior." Furthermore, in Fraser's view, recognition through the remediation of subordinate social status has the potential to transform wider social patterns of representation, interpretation, and communication because it goes beyond the limited demand of identity politics that a group's "cultural specificity" be acknowledged (Benhabib 2002, 70).

While Fraser's and others' concerns about the dominance of identity-based recognition seem fair, it's not clear to me that her solution doesn't create problems of its own. Although formally the status model does not reject culturally mediated harms to a group, it certainly seems to downplay them. (That dismissal of "free-floating cultural representations or discourses" is a bit sweeping.) A more fundamental difficulty is that, as so often happens in debates about disability, it holds up "participatory parity" (Fraser 2000) as a normative ideal. Fraser's model of social justice works for those disabled people for whom equal opportunity for social and economic participation is a highly desirable goal (see Danermark and Gellerstedt 2004), but it glosses over the fact that there are types of impairment that render participatory *parity* out of the question, though not of course participation of other kinds and degrees. Little thought is given in this model to whether attempts "to establish the subordinated party as a full partner in social life" leave out (and therefore effectively render invisible) all those disabled people for whom equality of participation is not of highest priority.

A COLLECTIVE DISABILITY IDENTITY?

To claim that disability can be a political identity is to go a few steps further than the more diffuse concept of a disability community, to which I will

return in a moment. The concept of a political activity based on group identity instead of ideology or a project of reform is historically recent, and
many of its parameters are still unclear. Identity-based politics refers to
groups that are formed not through the exercise of free choice assumed by
liberal democracy, but through an *unchosen characteristic* such as gender or
disability (Kenny 2004, 4). Now this is a harder distinction to hold firm
than first appears. While one may have no choice at all in the label one is
given by others, to deliberately take up a stake in the fortunes of women or
disabled people is a different act, with a different set of consequences, from
recognizing that one is a woman or has an impairment. Moreover, membership of a group based on an unchosen characteristic can nevertheless
sometimes be avowed or denied quite easily, so that it more closely resem-
bles an association by choice. Being Swiss is different from being a woman
because in principle it is possible to give up Swiss nationality,[2] while it is
not possible—or not nearly as possible—to stop being a woman. On the
other hand, critics of political liberalism, especially feminists, have questioned the accuracy of liberalism's model of associative groups, in particular the assumption that our belonging to these groups is a matter of free, rational, conscious choice. Many of the groups we belong to are neither
purely found nor purely chosen, but the result of a complex mixture of
choice, accident, habit, availability (does the group exist at all?), and so on.

Despite some fuzziness, though, these identity groupings can be distinguished from traditional, voluntary political associations. And the idea of
responding politically to unchosen particularities of identity sits uneasily
with a classic reading of liberal democracy in which features like your gender or ethnicity, or whether you can walk or not, are irrelevant to civil status. Identity politics asserts collective identities on the very features that the
liberal tradition does not consider to fall within the political realm. The
novel feature of identity politics is that the demand is not for inclusion or
respect "'in spite of' one's differences. Rather, what is demanded is respect
for oneself as different" (Kruks 2001, 85). Kwame Anthony Appiah suggests
that the liberal desire for universalization is in a sense driven by the awareness that it's easier to treat as an equal someone who has been "dis-
encumbered of attributes" that might otherwise compromise our respect for
them—disvalued attributes like impairments, for instance (2004, xv).

In fact, for identity-based politics as generally understood, the demand is
not simply for inclusion or respect, but for remediation as well. Identity
groups organize around the claim that they have been subjected to social injustice because of the features that mark them out. Formulated this way, it is
clear that two sets of issues are involved. The first has to do with the validity
of the claim to injustice and the form that any restitution should take. These
issues are normally best resolved through considering empirical evidence relating to the claim and public negotiation about compensation. A second set

of issues has to do with the validity of the group identity being claimed (Young 1990). At a minimum, having an identity-based politics suggests that there is some sort of collective identity to start with. Although some emergent political identities are of the kind we are already used to seeing *as* a group (ethnicities or national identities, regional groups, religions, linguistic or cultural groupings), the real difficulties arise with unfamiliar, more contested social categories such as gender, sexuality, gender identity, or disability. Delineating political identity is tricky for the more novel groupings that have not yet become socially entrenched and cannot rest on precedent, and disability presents a particularly hard case for identity arguments because of the disagreement about the background theory of disability.

A central objection to disability identity politics, then, is that claiming any kind of collective disability identity, whether politically or in a broader cultural sense, is meaningless because of the lack of clarity, both inside and outside the group, about what its members have in common. The more somatically and medically inclined theoretical perspectives on disability will see commonality in phenotypic deviation itself, perhaps most clearly in particular impairment groups—visual or hearing impairments, mobility impairments, and so on (Watson 2002). In this case disability identity and its politics will then refer to those people whose bodies deviate more than an accepted amount from the norm. Given the difficulty of unambiguously defining limits to phenotypic normality, though, impairment per se probably does not measure up as a sound basis for a shared political identity. Adherents to the strong social model, on the other hand, will suggest that the common feature of a political disability identity is not any kind of impairment, but the experience of oppression. Yet as we saw earlier, second-wave disability theorists question the universality of either *oppression* or *discrimination* as the invariant disability attribute. Disabled people undergo a wide range of experiences connected with their impairment, not all of which can easily be labelled as oppression. Sometimes redescription will allow events to be reconfigured: not being able to follow the television program because it has no subtitles may need to be redescribed as a disabling barrier before it can be recognized as having anything in common with the lack of wheelchair-accessible restaurants. Often, though, disabled people want to include in their identity *as* disabled other instances of exclusion, rejection, or isolation, and also more positive experiences, which are harder to collect under a blanket term of oppression.

So some critics worry that the only way a disability identity can be made to exist is by essentializing and homogenizing experiences that are more contingent and diverse. These are criticisms that have parallels within the wider debates of poststructuralist feminism and cultural theory of the late twentieth and early twenty-first centuries. The Foucauldian critique says that disability politics is trying to make ontological an identity that is in fact produced by

disciplinary regimes of practices and discourses (Morrow 2004, 278). Analysts
of political cultures for their part concentrate more on the risk that internal divergence and dissent are being smoothed away for the convenience of being
able to treat disabled people, theoretically and bureaucratically, as a unit. According to theorists like Benhabib, for instance, there is no group, community,
or culture—not even the ones that we tend to think of as coherent—that is a
clearly definable whole. Rather, these entities are "complex human practices of
signification and representation, of organization and attribution, which are internally riven by conflicting narratives" (2002, ix). She identifies a general tendency to lapse into false reification and homogenization and blames it on
what she calls a "reductionist sociology of culture" (4) that is driven to present
all communities and cultures as neater than they really are. The trap of denying the ragbag reality, however, is that in the end few people can recognize
themselves or their communities in these tidied-up descriptions. And indeed,
empirical research has shown that people with impairments who are hesitant
about claiming the identity of "disabled" for their own may do so because the
politically idealized version of it fails to speak to their condition.

Cultural theorists who take this approach tend to locate the problem in
the outsiders to a culture. Outsiders are more inclined to impose a false coherence, whether in the attempt to understand the awkward reality or for
the less desirable political purpose of controlling it. From within, its members are better placed to see (they may be unable to avoid seeing) the frac-
ture lines of internal diversity and conflict (Kenny 2004, 101). These critics,
however, often make the complementary mistake of idealizing the epistemic and ethical purposes of the group itself. They miss the fact that some
of the group's *own* members may prefer to project an image of coherence,
for overtly political reasons; this seems to be what has happened in parts of
the disability movement. As the strong social model organizes disability
identity primarily around the experience of oppression, it is possible that
people with impairment who do not perceive themselves as oppressed are
not seen as disabled or are told they have a false consciousness and are in
denial about the realities of their lives. "Disability identity" focused on the
consciousness of material oppression becomes the only *valid* form of collective identification.

As well as questioning the empirical validity of organizing disability identity solely around oppression or discrimination, some disability scholars
are also unwilling to take impairment as the only characteristic of relevance
in a nuanced theory of disability identity. These critics argue that other axes
of identification are always present, intersecting to modulate the experience
of impairment, and at times taking precedence in terms of subjectivity. The
political claims and goals of disability activism need to be modified in order to reflect this fragmented reality. For many people with impairment
there will be periods of their lives when the defining features of their iden-

tity, and/or the community to which they want to prioritize allegiance, will be (say) being a father, or a postal worker, or Sri Lankan, and not necessarily being disabled. Susan Peters writes that after a time of almost unidimensional commitment to the disability movement, "I began to feel the need to re/define myself as an individual and to validate my personal biography of unique lived experiences in multiple communities—only one of which was my disability network" (2000, 215).

Contemporary sociological evidence suggests that most people are more accurately regarded as participating in more than one social identity, and in our daily lives we are skilled at negotiating the constant shifts in their salience. Consequently, any theory of common political cause around identity must take into account that groups are made up of people with multiple, simultaneous, and sometimes noncontinuous commitments and allegiances (Whitebrook 2001, 137). There is little to be gained and a lot to be lost in clinging doggedly to an idea of the place impairment *ought* to hold in disabled people's lives, if there is good empirical evidence and theoretical arguments that it doesn't. However, acknowledging that identification with disability is not always primary in disabled people's lives does not render the identification that does happen, to the degree it does, morally or politically insignificant. To argue that would mean that an identity has to override all others, at all times, in order to count, and this is not true for most people. With increasing recognition that no subject's identity may be explained wholly in terms of one category, recent work in disability studies has begun to explore the experience of impairment from within other minority perspectives such as feminism (Fine and Asch 1988; Wendell 1996; Meekosha 1998; Fawcett 2000), ethnicity (Ahmad 2000; Hussain 2005; Hernandez 2005), and sexual orientation (Shakespeare et al. 1996; Clare 1999; Whitney 2006).

Ironically, to act as if disability is always and inevitably the master identity that overwhelms all others echoes the "sin of synecdoche" that Adrienne Asch and David Wasserman diagnose among people who choose to screen for abnormalities prenatally and terminate on the basis of them (2005). In their view, prenatal selection and similar selective practices make the error of allowing one piece of information (one of the few that is available about the future human at that stage) to stand for the whole life. Taking only one axis of identification to account for every aspect of a person's subjectivity is a similar sort of error. Just as in the example of prenatal selection, when impairment is present it comes to stand for the whole, overriding other characteristics with an ease that reveals much about our cultural ambivalence toward phenotypic difference.

In addition to the objection that a collective disability identity is an oversimplified fiction, some cultural critics see strong political identity claims as having a potentially disastrous "normative thrust." According to Appiah,

"Demanding respect for people as blacks and as gays requires that there are some scripts that go with being an African-American or having same sex desires. There will be proper ways of being black and gay, there will be expectations to be met, demands to be made" (1994, 162–63). Historically the parameters of "proper ways of being disabled" have been imposed by outsiders to that state rather than by disabled people themselves. But growing political self-assertion and the concomitant desire to have a coherent identity to bring into the political arena increases the likelihood that the same pressures of expectation operate within the group itself. To some observers the disability movements in the UK and United States have already gone some way toward developing inflexible ways of being disabled, or to paraphrase Moya Lloyd on women, "establishing what is or is not permissible for [disabled people] to be and do" (Lloyd 2005, 25). For a disabled person to be found authentic within that discourse she must present in a recognizable way or risk having her claim to belonging rejected and so lose out on the material, psychic, and moral benefits of being able to invoke disability as part of her own narrative of identity.

It may be argued that even if ontological or epistemological coherence is not empirically true, it is strategically necessary in order to advance the political program for disabled people, just as Gayatri Spivak famously claimed that a strategic essentialism is/was a necessary temporary stage for the women's movement (Spivak 1990a). Among the counterarguments that can be called on here, one could question the practical and psychic feasibility of taking up an oversimplified, in effect knowingly false, framework for identity and then putting it down again once it has served its purpose. (Who knows when it has served its purpose? Whose purpose has it then served? And who, exactly, is doing the taking up and putting down?) The political question is whether something like a strategic essentialism is useful in achieving a group's goals; and the answer might be that it is, in the political arena and in the short term. But whatever its practical advantages, essentialism does not sit comfortably in areas, like academic work, that depend on sensitivity to complexity and nuance. And it is also difficult to see how such a strategy can be even politically viable in the longer term, if it is wilfully epistemically inaccurate and therefore, for all the reasons discussed earlier, undermines the moral subjectivity of at least some disabled people.

A final objection that collective disability identity faces is the accusation that it is bad for you. Identity politics involves people staking a claim to a shared history of structural oppression or disadvantage. Some commentators reason that any group that owes its existence to historical or current grievance inevitably develops a pathology of ingrained victimhood. Individual group members may be psychologically damaged by the incorporation of victimhood as a key constituent of their identities. People who have done this, it is argued, are then unable to eradicate the part of a victim from their self-concepts. They will be trapped in the role of victim, and (it is further argued) this is a bad thing because whatever else it does psychologically, to see oneself as perpetually hard done by is destructive to one's capacity to act as a competent, self-determining moral agent. And whatever it does to the individual, there is a parallel fear that collectively, a group identity with grievance at its core sets a pattern for an inevitable "politics of recrimination and rancour" (Brown 1993, 390). If the group only exists through its claim for compensation and/or its constant vigilance for ongoing oppression, then in order to justify the existence of a group in which its members have so much invested, compensation must always be inadequate and oppression and disadvantage must always be found.

These are complex arguments and they need fuller treatment than I can give them here. However, there are some strong initial responses that can be made. One is that sometimes, a sense of victimhood is absolutely correct. Being or having been a victim of injustice can be a factually sound description of one's life. There is certainly a risk of its becoming the *only* description that one has, and most of us have encountered people whose unremitting attachment to being hard done by corrodes their own lives as much as it alienates everyone else. But to be denied ownership of the experience of being victimized, or to be pushed to adopt the life narrative of "survivor" when that does not jibe with one's subjective knowledge, must be just as destructive to one's self-trust. Hence, for a period of time that will vary with person and circumstance, claiming a sense of victimhood can be morally helpful because it asserts the right to say what is true about one's own life narrative. Saying "for a time" implies something else: people do not inevitably become forever entrenched in the role of victim in the way that is being suggested. Certainly it is a possibility, but not, I would think, an overwhelming one, and the likelihood is further reduced by adopting a model of collective identity in which disability coexists dynamically with identities rooted in other communities in which one is *not* a victim.

The perpetuation of *collective* victimhood, on the other hand, seems to me much more probable. For one thing, once any social grouping becomes widely recognized, it is locked in place by a scaffolding of institutional forces (political, economic, and so on) that are no longer under the control of its members. Nondisabled people make their own professional and emotional investments in keeping alive the disability identity that *they* recognize, which may not accurately reflect the evolving realities of disabled people's experience. One way of guarding against this would be to ensure that the political identity of disabled people is not solely about the redress of current grievance and compensation for historical wrong, however important these things are. Both the strong social model and the civil rights–based model seem to me intrinsically more likely to encourage a dependence on injustice as the *raison d'être* of the political organization of disability. Versions of social-relational models may have greater theoretical space in which a collective identity can emerge in the commonalities of embodied engagements with the world: engagements that are distinctive because they involve phenotypic variation, but not inevitably injustice or oppression.

COLLECTIVE IDENTITY AND TRANSFORMATION

Given the problems of defining disability identity at all, and the potential for some versions of disability identity to distort moral perception and agency rather than enhance it, is it still possible to view collective identification as helpful to disabled people's moral subjectivity? I think it is. Collective political self-identification has been a major factor (though not the only one) in bringing about change for the better in the social and economic status of disabled people over the last century. The opening up of education, work, and social support has had enormously positive and very tangible effects on disabled people's exercise of choice and capacity for self-determination. However, tracing how political identification has helped do this (and why it has not done more) is not my concern here. I want to concentrate on the potential of collective political identification and action to transform how disabled people make sense of their lives, and hence their capacity to act as moral as well as political subjects. The separation here is an analytic one—as the models of identity politics that tie redistribution to recognition demonstrate, the social/psychological and the economic/political dimensions of culture are inevitably interdependent. But it helps to keep in view the point that collective identification has effects on potential moral agency that are not visible in obvious political action.

The politics of recognition is not just about being accepted as a player on the political terrain, but about processes of self-definition. The previous chapter showed how redescribing what one has experienced as a disabled person around alternative narratives can be very powerful. Many personal accounts by disabled people attest to the impact of redescription that involves a conscious alignment of one's life with the political disability movement, and often, because of the particular form taken by the disabled people's movement in the UK, United States, and Australasia, this has also meant redescription in the terms of a narrative of struggle against social marginalization. I am not going to repeat here the benefits to self-concept that this can have: Robert Murphy, a disabled sociologist, put it succinctly many years ago when he wrote that "the most lasting benefits of any struggle against perceived oppression are not the tangible gains but the transformations of consciousness of the combatants" (Murphy 1987, 157).

This makes the point that identity politics is productive as well as reflective of the political subject. I started this discussion of disability identity politics from the commonplace view that there needs to be a group (a collective identity) first, in order for it to make political claims about injustices. This is a model of identity politics that sees it expressing the demands of a preconstituted identity (Lloyd 2005, 36) made up of characteristics that the individual disabled person shares with others. Subjectivity is a capacity that subjects *have*, and which they then exercise in the moral, political, and social orders. There are contemporary accounts of subjectivity, however, that offer alternative ways of looking at moral and political agency and the role of political identification in it. Rejecting a model of the subject as unitary or stable, or existing before it is brought into speech, many poststructuralist theorists would say that political identity is best thought of as an effect of politics rather than its source. Moya Lloyd, for example, roundly criticizes feminist identity politics for reversing its order of priority (39), saying that feminists who draw on concepts of identity "have tended to conceive of it in constative terms" as expressing who women are in terms of pregiven attributes or experiences (38). In other words, and counter to the idea that all disabled people share an identity that is the basis for the legitimacy of disability politics, poststructuralists like Lloyd would see the disabled self as having no ontological status of its own, but as being performatively produced through political acts.

We may not want to follow the poststructuralist argument quite this far, and in chapter 1 I discussed why I find its sidelining of prediscursive embodied identity particularly unhelpful for understanding the experience of disabled bodies. Attempts to theorize moral and political subjects tend to settle around one of the two extremes, which may be categorized as modernist possessors of agency on the one hand, and epiphenomena of discourses on the other. Each model of agency is able to provide explanations that are compelling for some behaviors of the subject but implausible for others. For the sake of this discussion I propose the moderate, although perhaps less rhetorically satisfying, compromise that cultural and political identity is consolidated through the struggle for recognition even if it is not created by it. I do not want to follow Lloyd and Butler in taking the operation of agency to be prior, that is, to demand that it generates either the subject or the collective, but instead suggest a more dialectical and recursive process between identity and acts of agency.

This both/and compromise nevertheless has some important implications for the ethics of recognition. If a minority identity first exists and then makes a claim for recognition, the moral harm that Charles Taylor and others see here lies in denying recognition to the self of what it *is*, and therefore hampering its expression of agency *as* that preexisting self. Lloyd and other poststructuralists would want to place more emphasis on the idea that at least part of the harm of nonrecognition comes from denying a group the social space in which to make the political and moral claims that are a necessary part of the emergence of the collective identity itself. From this point of view, the argument which is sometimes used—that the notion of disability identity did not exist before some disabled people decided to invent it—is not a criticism, but rather a description of the process by which all social identities appear. In Ian Hacking's words, "Numerous kinds of human beings and human acts come into being hand in hand with our invention of categories labelling them" and the social or political activities that represent the category as real (1986, 236).

The transformative effect of generating novel "kinds of human beings," however, goes beyond the self-consciousness of the group. That is to say, collective political identification acts not only on disabled people's own understandings of the moral significance of impairment, but on nondisabled society's interpretations of it as well. Nancy Fraser, as we saw, wants to distinguish what she defines as the politics of recognition from identity politics, arguing that the goals of recognition should be more socially ambitious than just helping a group affirm its identity. A politics of recognition could aim to change "societal patterns of representation, interpretation and communication in ways that would change everyone's social identity," not just the self-identification of disabled people (Fraser and Honneth 2003, 13). Plainly, this is a more ambitious ethical program than identity politics is commonly conceived of having. But it would be more in line with the voices of the disability movement who argue that true recognition of disability requires a radical reengineering of the frames of reference through which we understand normal bodies and normal social organization.

RECLAIMING DISABILITY COMMUNITY

I would want to conclude from all this that a form of collective identity offers moral as well as political benefits to disabled people. Against that must be balanced the drawbacks of identity politics that threaten to, and sometimes do, compromise the benefits. One key difficulty here is that the term "identity" is being forced to do too much work: symbolic, descriptive, political, and ethical. In addition to identity's being a focus around which political activity can assemble, it has to offer a social reality, and a framework for personal self-understanding that can be incorporated into the narratives of individual identity too. Sometimes the imperatives of these various tasks come into conflict, such as when the need to present a uniform voice on the political stage runs up against the awkwardly incoherent reality of disabled people's lives.

The worst of these conflicts might possibly be avoided by heading in the direction Fraser indicated, separating the domains of identity formation and political recognition. However, rather than jettison the hope of a collective disability identity altogether, an alternative would be to reclaim the notion of the "disability community." Although a vaguer and superficially less rigorous concept than identity politics, community could be usefully retained as a way of talking about identity that runs in parallel with a narrower politics of recognition focusing on social position. By "community" here I mean nothing more complex than a collection of people who perceive some commonality of experience with and shared responsibility for each other. It's possible to consider yourself part of such a community without necessarily feeling that the group is obliged to make claims on the political and economic institutions of civil society. As we have seen, not everyone is convinced that disabled people share enough elements of experience and enough self-consciousness of difference from nondisabled people for the language of community to ring true. Disabled experience is varied, and if there is such a thing as a disabled community, it is a mix of found and chosen, on a sliding scale depending on impairment and circumstances. For impairments that are present at birth or early childhood, it is possible to identify with others who have related impairments, through shared experiences in special schools, clinics, and so on. For most impairments, though, this does not happen, especially not if children (or their parents) are unfamiliar with impairment or resist being associated with it (Morris 1991, 37). When impairment comes later in life, a person may find it hard to see it as constituting much of a commonality with all other disabled people. Effectively, while some people with impairment are satisfied to consider themselves part of a disability community, even one that is more conceptual (or virtual) than material, others would strongly reject any notion of there being such a community at all, and yet others would acknowledge its existence but deny that they were part of it (see Watson 2002; Ville et al. 2003). Still, there are those who do claim that the common experience of being different, other, liminal, negatively marked by phenotypic variation in ways that are not equivalent to being gendered or raced, is enough to deserve the term "community" (Peters 2000; Hernandez 2005). The point about community is that it can operate with a more flexible, looser range of individual disability identities, and more contested moral understandings, than political identity can.

Disability is an anomalous, marginal social status, and therefore any community of disabled people will also be anomalous and marginal. By definition such a community is a carrier of heterodox epistemic and moral views (mixed in with more orthodox ones). The process of political recognition and self-generation, then, involves more than acknowledging the emergence of a collective identity. A disability community should also be the place that reframes emergent identities more positively, redescribing disabled subjects and their lives in their own terms rather than anyone else's. The community that undertakes such acts of redescription in defiance of prevailing norms forms what Cheshire Calhoun (1989) has called an abnormal moral context. The epistemic advantage of the group prises open and makes explicit the gap between the behavior prescribed by the majority society and the lived reality of the minority group. It's this process of restructuring and reinterpreting one's experience that generates a new version of subjectivity, owned collectively and individually. The disability community then provides the *base* for the political claim for recognition, but the identities fostered within the community have permission to be more multiple, fragmented, and even contradictory than the voice of a political project can afford to be. By relocating the responsibility to embody and articulate collective disability identity to the community, the political renegotiation of status and resources is freed from the obligation to express everything there is to say about disability identity. It can also help guard against a distorted view of collective agency as only effected in politically visible actions. Just as individual moral agency is not solely about obvious choices and acts, but also includes the interior capacities for reflection and discernment, collective moral agency is expressed through the working out of identities that resist existing morally harmful ascriptions. Collective moral agency operates too in renegotiating the everyday social background against which progressive political choice and action become possible.

There is a further reason for retaining or reclaiming the idea of a "community" in disability discourse. Communities have a different kind of moral significance that is not strictly to do with gaining political recognition. (It can be, but doesn't have to be.) Communities have their own narratives of identity that contain their history and are key sources of shared moral understanding. Both found and chosen communities operate within structures of implicit and explicit moral norms, and their members are likely to turn to them for guidance. While this is sometimes done consciously (a Catholic pacifist might mine her religious tradition to help form her opinion about just war, for example), social and moral psychology suggest that far more often those norms are cognitively internalized at levels that are not accessible to consciousness, at least not without effort. Hence the nature of the authority of these moral norms is perceived differently according to the nature of the group.

So too is the nature of the bonds between members of the group. "Community" implies a distinctive pattern of responsibilities and solidarities that is not the same as the pattern associated with "group" or "collective." We speak of communities rather than groups at times when we want to convey the idea that the bonds between members are something more than a contract between rational decision makers. Bonds like these can involve unknown others. In a survey of university students with disabilities, for instance, Olney and Brockelman (2003) found that even students who professed not to identify with the disability rights movement felt that as disabled people they had experiences that were not available to most people, and they also felt a responsibility to share their experiences, knowledge, and strategies with others. Similarly, authors of disability memoirs, like those discussed in the previous chapter, are motivated in part by their need for self-expression, but also by something like a sense of duty to others. Community ties may also be strongly affective bonds. They reflect the asymmetry of dependencies of a community in a way that is not the case for the vocabulary of group or association. The language of community carries a greater consciousness of mutual responsibility, with all the benefits and burdens that entails. When we talk about a chosen community, the "choice" refers to the decision (to the degree that it is a decision) to become part of it, not about whether one accepts the moral responsibilities that go along with membership; these are, or should be, nonnegotiable.

Distinguishing the "community" and the "political" dimensions of collective disability identity helps separate out the different although overlapping moral functions the two ideas perform. A theory of two processes does not give a complete description of the ways in which disabled subjectivities are formed or the conditions for social and political change generated. But it has the advantage, I believe, of maximizing the ethical benefits that the different operations of collective identity provide. A disability community will ideally provide a social and cultural space in which a wide repertoire of identity narratives can be developed. As a "morally abnormal" community it especially offers a heterodox context in which more epistemically truthful, morally sustaining descriptions of disabled lives can be formed, and in doing so it provides social and psychological support to the widest variety of disabled people. Ideally again, political disability activity helps rearrange social status and redistribute material and cultural resources for the benefit of disabled people. By not being tied to the promotion of particular identity claims, however, it maximizes its political efficacy and avoids the trap of setting up too limited a range of disability identities as normative.

It may in any case be a mistake to look for a model of collective disability identity that does not also contain collective *dis*agreement. As we have seen, there are ethical and epistemological dangers associated with forcing coherence where there is none. Benhabib says that being fixated on achieving internal coherence risks missing important ethical points: "In a world without conflict, questions of justice . . . are held at bay" (2002, 57). She goes so far as to suggest that effort should be redirected away from attempts to define cultural identities, and toward locating sites of dissonance, inside and outside the culture, where ethical and political shift can best occur. Many political and cultural theorists have taken the view that dissonances, the bits that don't fit, are necessary for psychic, political, and social change, triggered by (depending on theory) the symptomatic expression of unconscious conflict, the emergence of contradiction through a Gramscian counterhegemonic discourse, or a Foucauldian analysis exposing the sites in present social arrangements where conditions are optimal for change. Thus in one narrative of second-wave feminism, internal conflicts over the true meaning of feminist identity fatally undermine its political credibility. But in another, the internal faults and fractures are precisely those points where women's agency is most readily to be found. For Spivak (1990b) this is the "practical politics of the open end," in which conflicts between those involved are recognized as not only inevitable but as the basis from which new narratives of political structure are generated. So the pressing ethical question for disability identity becomes whether enough flexibility can be built into the ways of having/being/expressing impairment to enable the kind of transformative social shifts that many disability activists think is necessary; and if such shifts are as subtle as the model suggest, how do we identify accurately whether in fact these shifts take us in the direction we want to go, or take us in a more conservative, even morally harmful direction that we would want to avoid at all costs?

THE REALITY OF COLLECTIVE IDENTITY

In practice, arguing whether or not a collective disability identity exists, what kind of identity it is, and how it fits into one or another theoretical framework, is beside the point. The weight of experiential and empirical evidence is that some form of collective identity has already been effective: the emergence of "disability" as an organizing concept and of "disabled people" as a political grouping so closely parallels improvements in disabled people's social and economic status that it is impossible to deny a relationship, albeit not entirely straightforward, between the two (Campbell and Oliver 1996; Shakespeare 2006). There is also some evidence that the growing profile of disability activism has changed the forms of identification that disabled people use. Darling (2003) suggests that the typology of "adaptations" that she originally devised in 1979 is being gradually supplemented, although not yet supplanted, by an affirmation model in which disability can be a positive social identity rather than something that needs to be normalized as far as possible. She hypothesizes that although the affirmation model is becoming more established, particularly among a subgroup of parents and disabled people who accept alternative norms of ability and appearance, there is a risk of creating a split between these politically right-on people and others who prefer to go along with prevailing norms. She also—and this brings me back to the point I have been making throughout this book—regrets the lack of data with which to answer relatively straightforward questions about "the actual identities of people with disabilities today" (Darling 2003, 884). If some *form of* a collective disability identity makes a significant difference to the lives of some disabled people, a bioethics that takes disability seriously needs to take note of it, as part of its empirical work of grasping actual moral understandings, and also to identify ways of bringing the opinions of disabled people into bioethical discourse.

NOTES

1. Note that this work tends not to distinguish between the recognition as a political entity of a group that was previously socially recognized but disvalued, such as feminists, and that of a collective that was not previously recognized as a group at all. Recent examples of the latter include sexual minorities as well as disabled people. The parallel for individual subjectivity would be the difference between replacing toxic narratives of identity and generating missing ones—see chapter 6.
2. The Swiss might be puzzled as to why anyone should want to.

8

All Clues and (Some) Solutions[1]

One cannot overestimate the role of epistemic and discursive manipulation in understanding how flawed, even vicious, moral orders are reproduced.

—Margaret Urban Walker

What would a deeper engagement with the experience of disability bring to bioethics? And what might bioethical thinking about disability then bring to disability studies, and to disabled people?

This book is an argument for more empirically and experientially grounded bioethical work on impairment and disability. I first suggested that up to now, bioethics has primarily taken an ethics of disability approach to impairment. It has considered the ethical stance that we, where *we* means the nondisabled majority, should take theoretically toward impairment, and concretely toward disabled people in our society. Bioethics does this in the context of considering biomedical interventions that have especial relevance to disabled people: preeminently prenatal or preimplantation diagnosis at the start of life, therapeutic or normalizing interventions in the course of life, and decisions about treating or withholding treatment in illness or at the end of life. An ethics of disability approach to these and similar questions comes naturally to bioethics for several reasons, but among them is that working bioethicists[2] often have no first-person experience of impairment. They may be as unaware of the need to be better informed about it as they are of the sources that would do so. It should be clear by now that I think the range of approaches bioethics has so far brought to bear on disability is depressingly small. I have argued that we need the insights of many other disciplines in order to map out the empirical and experiential realities of living with an impairment before we can legitimately undertake ethical judgments that weigh up the desirability of those lives, or calculate the cost/benefit balance of interventions that we hope will improve them. Judgments about quality of life or permissible interventions stand a higher chance of being mistaken, and therefore of being unjust, if they are made on the basis of inadequate knowledge. This isn't just bad luck: there is an ethical fault here if we recognize that our knowledge is inadequate (and I have provided evidence that it is), and that there are ways of filling in the gaps (which there are), and we still persist in making those ethical judgments.

I have also argued that to address the gaps in our understanding bioethics needs more than just empirical data. The subjective experience of disabled people is a necessary part of grasping what it is like to live as/in an impaired embodiment. Phenomenological accounts of the experience of impairment are not as easy to get at as empirical data; nor is it straightforward to integrate them into the bioethical database. But if bioethicists want to be able to say that the *bad thing* about disability, the experienced disadvantage of it, is sufficient grounds for morally serious medical interventions, then we need evidence that the disadvantage is as great as is claimed. Many (although I emphasize, not all) disabled people would say that the disadvantage of their impairment is *not* as bad; or that the disadvantage is not the impairment itself, but something else, such as the experience of exclusion or being treated as a freak; or that while some elements of the impairment are absolutely unwanted, others are more benign; or that the experience is such a formative part of their identity that they cannot think of it as a disadvantage at all; and so on. Much of what I've said concerns the moral significance of disability as identity constituting. In *Moral Contexts* (2003), Margaret Urban Walker identifies deep relationships, social roles, personal ideals, constitutive projects, and group loyalties as being identity constituting (6). She excludes physical traits, and here I disagree: I have been arguing that phenotypic variation *is* identity constituting, in varying degrees.

To claim that bioethical analysis would benefit from greater input from experiences of impairment and disability implies that there is something about those experiences which might make a difference to moral evaluation. It suggests that the experience of phenotypic variation can modify moral understandings, in obvious and more subtle ways. As I've said before, taking this line does not presuppose that embodied variation *does* lead to observable differences in moral understandings, but only that it *might*; and if so, that the differences are likely to be complex, to operate on numerous levels, and to require more than one methodology to identify them. In four chapters at the heart of this book I considered possible analytical approaches to teasing out those differences in terms of prediscursive, presocial somatic experience, the embodied interaction of the self and the social world, and the development of personal identity and political identification. Just before that, in the discussion of moral epistemology in chapter 3, I raised the problem of normativity.

NORMATIVITY

Suppose it turns out to be the case that embodied variation leads to differences in somatic, psychic, or social experience such that people's moral understandings are changed. Both bioethicists and disability theorists might find themselves united (for once) in asking the question, what difference does that make to the normative work we do? Along with many feminist ethicists and empirically inclined bioethicists, I take ethics to be an enterprise with a larger empirical component than has been recognized. In line with this view, I've been putting forward a case for a naturalized bioethical epistemology as the basis of a disability bioethics. But however much recognition there is of ethics' empirical side, most moral philosophers and bioethicists would want to maintain that the *raison d'être* of bioethics is its normative role. How, they ask, does expanding empirical and experiential knowledge help bioethicists reach normative conclusions about moral acts or agents? Knowing more about other individuals', groups', or cultures' practices and points of view expands our epistemic purchase on morally troubling situations, but it does not tell us whether they are good practices or good points of view to hold.

Moral philosophers generally want to stand firm against any equivalence of descriptive and normative statements. They view the introduction of empirical and experiential data as at best irrelevant to ethics' normative force, and at worst guilty of diluting it. Edmund Pellegrino exemplifies this position when he says that "neither descriptive ethics nor analytical-metaethical inquiry can establish what is morally good, right, or required in a particular case. They cannot extrapolate from the 'is' to the 'ought' without destroying normative ethics" (1995, 162). Caution about abdicating ethics' normative responsibility is not confined to mainstream bioethics, however; feminist and other bioethicists at the social and disciplinary margins also find it troubling, as they want to keep hold of the capacity to set normative boundaries that define some attitudes and behaviors toward women or minorities as morally wrong, irrespective of whether they happen to be endorsed by a particular community. And similarly, disability ethics wants to retain the idea that some attitudes and behaviors toward disabled people are morally wrong, even if the majority community endorses them (as historically has often been the case).

Neither bioethics nor disability studies, then, can abandon its normative responsibilities. What both bioethicists and disability scholars want is for the additional epistemic resources to make normative claims about impairment *better*. A minimal contribution would be simply to provide a more complete, accurate, and insightful description of morally troubling situations. Even bioethicists who would not describe themselves as empirically oriented are likely to agree that context sensitivity helps to identify the "major problems actually faced" and how they are dealt with (Nelson 2000b), or how best to implement healthcare policies and so on in real life. Indeed, some projects of empirical ethics have the stated aim of improving a given healthcare practice and providing normative guidelines for the future. In this minimalist usage, empirical information helps to flesh out the description of the morally troubling situation, reducing the risk of injustice arising out of ignorance or lack of thought. Moral evaluation still takes place from the usual perspective of the observer, who is not required to make any empathic or imaginative steps toward entering the experience of another. In fact, as we saw earlier, the perspective of the bioethical observer is routinely taken as epistemically delocalized. Throughout this book, however, I have been advocating the need to go beyond the sheer acquisition of data, helpful though that is, and to try to comprehend social contexts, including the contexts of academic bioethics or disability activism, as the places where moral understandings are developed and played out. Becoming better informed about the situation or problem *as seen by* people with various impairments, parents of disabled children, or prospective parents of embryos with genetic lesions does more than add useful detail to the analytic picture. It provides a different picture, from a different place, for the exercise of normative analysis.

CRITICAL BIOETHICS

The critical approach to bioethics I introduced in chapter 3 (Hedgecoe 2004) takes a different approach to improving the quality of bioethical knowledge about disabled people's lives, and as a result does not fit as comfortably with bioethics' normative conventions as straightforwardly empirical methodologies. Critical bioethics converges with the older feminist tradition of ethical and bioethical critique exemplified in Walker's work on moral understanding, providing tools for examining the relationship between social power and the construction of knowledge—how the social organization of authority determines what it is possible for people to think. These analyses take the view that the standards of ethical evaluation can never be neutral or objective because they are generated within practices, discourses, and organizations that are themselves configured by relations of authority and dominance. According to Walker, such relationships of authority "allow some people to rig both [social-moral] arrangements and the perceptions of them, and so to obscure what is really happening to whom and why. It is this fund of knowledge that needs to be enlarged and theoretically articulated in general accounts and specific studies of *different relative moral positions in differentiated social lives"* (Walker 1998, 219; italics in original). "Specific studies" includes the lives of disabled people, not only because they are often unfamiliar to the majority nondisabled world, but because the new biotechnologies produce unprecedented *forms* of disabled living—the long-lived tetraplegic, the middle-aged person with cystic fibrosis, the cochlear implant wearer—which are socially and ethically unknown territory.

This is a form of scrutiny more familiar to the sociology of knowledge than bioethics (Ashcroft 2003), examining how particular issues become classified as respectively empirical or analytic, and how certain kinds of social inquiry are productive of the forms of life they set out to study. Empirical and other bioethical inquiry is best understood as a "sort of politics" (12), meaning that empirical bioethics must abandon any notion it has of itself as standing outside the exercise of power. This is a particular temptation for disability research, where the emancipatory roots of disability studies can lead its practitioners to believe that the gradient of power between researcher and researched has been leveled because of the politically progressive motives and democratic approach of the researcher (the power differential has gone because the researcher decides it has).

In the case of impairment, it is undeniable that mainstream bioethical analysis to date has sidestepped a lot of questions about the laws, institutions, and practices that facilitate the making of certain choices or adopting of certain attitudes. It is now quite commonplace for a Foucauldian analysis to hold up biomedical technology as the key contemporary area in which regimes of control and self-control are enacted, but so far this analysis has not been rigorously applied to questions of impairment and biopower (Tremain [2005] provides a notable exception). This is not a claim that disabled people are disproportionately subject to biomedical regulation and supervision—although that is often true—but rather that phenotypically variant people inevitably present a challenge to the conventions of embodiment and its regulation. Part of critical bioethics' task, then, is to scrutinize how cultural beliefs about the ontology and morality of impairment are simultaneously adopted and conveyed by the normative regulatory responses to phenotypic challenge.

To see the mode of inquiry as a normative practice in itself gives normativity a rather more ambiguous role than traditional moral philosophy would recognize. It follows a constructivist understanding of knowledge, in which the supposedly value-neutral approaches of empirical bioethics determine ahead of time which phenomena are worth observing, and what counts in the end as a result. A critical disability bioethics has the task of unraveling these predetermined normative framings, as far as it can from its *own* epistemological position, so that they are no longer taken for granted.

But acknowledging that social realities are more interwoven with moral lives and professional ethics than we once thought (or hoped) does not mean abandoning all attempts at ethical judgment. It is important not to conclude that conceding a level of epistemic authority to others means having to accept their moral narrative wholesale (Benhabib 2002, 7). A critical disability bioethics *examines* claims to moral authority based solely on personal experience of impairment, being a carer, being the sibling of a disabled person, or having professional expertise. That means that neither empirical data nor subjective accounts of experience have unconditional authority. Empirical research can be flawed, or biased, or start from the wrong questions. The beliefs that people hold because of their experience can be factually wrong or self-serving; some people may just lie.

Getting a better knowledge of contexts and experiences, then, may prompt morally significant shifts in how personal or group behavior is judged, but there must always be elements of morality that, because of the nature of human beings and societies, have to be retained. It is well beyond the scope of this chapter to put forward a case for any of the frameworks of widely applicable moral standards that have been proposed, historically or more recently. But few bioethicists or disability theorists are likely to find broadly sketched ethical frameworks unduly problematic; the problems, as we have seen, tend to arise when we try to fill in the outlines.

Today many social institutions, including healthcare and medical education, recognize the need to improve communication between ethnic and cultural groups. There are well-known examples (Anne Fadiman's *The Spirit Catches You and You Fall Down*, 1998, is one of them) of ethical firestorms flaring up when members of a culture with unfamiliar social-moral understandings of illness encounter the beliefs of Western biomedicine. Unlike these cultural confrontations, examples of misunderstanding and misrecognition around disability are generally much less obvious. In the main they involve subgroup(s) of people within one society sharing common moral foundations. They take the form of incomprehensible choices, or anomalous priorities, standing out against an otherwise unremarkable background of commonality. It is therefore improbable that disabled people will, by virtue of impairment, occupy *radically* different moral terrain from people without those impairments, any more than women occupy radically different terrain from men. What this means is that the significant differences that do exist are that much harder to spot. It also means that any differences cannot then be explained away as having been generated by a completely alien social-moral understanding.

This is not an argument for moral relativism of the sort that sees different groups or cultures as having incommensurable moral codes, but a particularism whereby, in different cases, similar acts have different consequences and meanings, and so may be evaluated differently. In each case we need to work out what matters to whom, and why it matters. Whatever the final judgment, all parties are likely to share some foundational moral concepts—about things like good, rights, welfare, safety, care, abandonment, cruelty, selfishness—even if what fills in the outlines of those concepts is the source of contention. The case of the "deaf babies by choice" is a good example of one fairly consistent moral understanding held by one fairly coherent group, enacted in behavior that ran counter to a different understanding held just as consistently by a different (hearing) group. The incompatibility between the culturally Deaf who see no disadvantage in having a child with hearing impairment and those who argue that parents have something like a duty to have the "best" possible child (see Savulescu 2001, 2007; Parker 2007) is generated within the moral knowledges held by these differently located people. Both culturally Deaf and hearing people nevertheless operate within a common social-moral framework that gives high value to the welfare of the child and of the community in which the family lives and also values giving (a restricted amount of) liberty to parents to make decisions on behalf of their children.

They differ in recognizing site-specific manifestations of these goods, and that makes a profound difference to the final conclusion. Here is the point where knowledge of other ways of being in the world has its effect. For the majority hearing community, it might turn out that knowing more about the Deaf world's structure, history, and future, and about the motivations and features of Deaf people's lives that make a preference "just obvious," would turn previously bizarre moral choices into more convincing ones. They might then agree that this is a morally permissible stance rather than an objectionable one. (They would probably still think that it is not generalizable, that is, that it would not be morally permissible for someone not embedded in the Deaf community to prefer a hearing-impaired child.) It might also be the case, of course, that Deaf people would shift their position with the benefit of greater knowledge of bioethicists' arguments against having a hearing-impaired child by choice. What needs to be remembered here, though, is that the epistemic bias and its effects are not symmetrical between majority and minority groups (Wendell 1996, 61).

So extending epistemic feelers into the experiences of unfamiliar phenotypes, or other unfamiliar ways of being, and becoming more critical of the sources of our own and others' ethical beliefs does not mean abandoning bioethics' essential task of identifying morally preferable ways of life and courses of action. It certainly does not mean, for example, that epistemic or ethical differences between disabled and nondisabled people are so great that any attempt at bridge building is not worth the effort. Exactly the opposite: the moral responsibility is to examine in breadth and depth how shareable knowledge can be identified. It does mean, as Walker says, that confirming the moral authority of our own and others' practices involves "discovering how they actually go, what they actually mean, and what it is actually like to live them from particular places within them" (2002, 110). In bioethics, this applies to practices that are continually being reshaped by the rapid advance of technologies. Testing moral authority in these cases clearly involves a lot more work than at present. Having come all this way, it may seem disappointing to have to conclude that an improved bioethical epistemology will not make bioethical judgments any easier. The hope, however, is that it will make them better.

BEYOND NORMATIVE BIOETHICS

Apart from refining bioethics' normative function, the exploration of disabled lives offers further benefits. In the remainder of this chapter I make some brief comments on its potential to (1) enlarge our understanding of foundational moral concepts, (2) affirm the role of bodies in moral life, (3) contribute to theorizing the ontological and moral meaning of disability, and (4) assert respect for moral subjectivity.

Disability, Autonomy, and Independence

Attention to impairment brings a much-needed fresh perspective to the philosophical concepts of autonomy, agency, dependence, and care. While the notion of autonomy is central to pretty much all Western moral and political philosophy, it has acquired a special status in medical and bioethics. The reasons for this are as much historical and pragmatic (to do with bioethics' support function to biomedicine) as theoretical. In Beauchamp and Childress' *Principles of Biomedical Ethics* (2001, first edition 1979) the text which structured the early development of the Anglo-American bioethics, ethical reasoning rests on the four central principles of autonomy, beneficence, nonmaleficence, and justice. All four principles are given as equal; over time, though, it has turned out that some principles are more equal than others, and in practice autonomy has attracted by far the most attention. It is no secret that not all bioethicists are happy about this. Some have reservations about the general preeminence of autonomy as an organizing principle,[3] while others are more worried by the ease with which autonomy is conflated with patients' freedom of choice, and respect for autonomy conflated with not blocking a patient's choice of treatment as long as it can be paid for.[4]

Moral and political philosophers continue to disagree on the characteristics of an autonomous agent, how one would recognize these characteristics in action, and whether truly autonomous agents exist at all. Nevertheless, although the theoretical formulations vary, they share a minimum consensus that autonomy has to do with personal *self-determination*. The subject who can be called autonomous has the capacity to imagine how she wants her life to go, and then to implement decisions to make it happen. Mainstream philosophy also agrees on some other features of autonomous agents that have been heavily criticized by feminists (Gilligan 1982; Baier 1985; Meyers 1989; Code 1991) as well as by communitarians and some postmodernist philosophers. The key features of these critiques are well known, and I won't labor them here. They all concern the characterization of the moral agent and the ways in which such an agent displays the features of autonomy. Although the theories of Kant, Mill, Rawls, and others are dissimilar, the critics say, they share a similar ideal of the autonomous moral agent as an atomistic, disembodied, rational, and unified locus of consciousness that is effectively interchangeable with other loci.[5] Critics reject these descriptions as flawed on the grounds that they leave out important features of the moral subject and of moral life. Any conception of autonomy draped around agents of this kind will be inadequate because in reality, agents are "emotional, embodied, desiring, creative, and feeling" as well as rational consciousnesses. Although modernist philosophy might treat them as interchangeable, they are "psychically internally differentiated and socially differentiated from others" (Mackenzie and Stoljar 2000, 21). The point is not that people *don't* make moral choices through a logical maximization of the benefits to themselves through reciprocal arrangements, but that they *also* behave as nonrational, emotional, embodied beings who are connected to others through ties of responsibility and dependence that are more often than not *non*reciprocal and not articulated. These features are constitutive of everyday moral life, at least as much as rational choices and agreements. So to set up an ideal of autonomous agency in which they are either ignored or characterized as regrettable flaws gives a misleading and depleted idea of moral subjectivity.

Feminist ethics and bioethics have been in the vanguard of crafting alternative models of autonomy. I've chosen to focus on relational autonomy here, because of the specific contribution it makes to thinking about disability and dependency. Relational autonomy holds that "persons are socially embedded" and that "agents' identities are formed within the context of social relationships and shaped by a complex of intersecting social determinants, such as race, class, gender, and ethnicity" (Mackenzie and Stoljar 2000, 4). Where mainstream perspectives broadly take autonomy to increase in linear proportion to a person's detachment from interpersonal obligations and ties, relational autonomy suggests that what actually makes autonomy possible is not detachment, but the social relationships that provide the conditions for experiencing and maintaining self-determination (Meyers 1989; Nedelsky 1989). A weak form of relational autonomy sees early social relationships as providing the ground for the later development of cognitive capacities needed for self-determination. Strong relational autonomy goes further, claiming that autonomy cannot even be conceived of outside a social context, because the activities that constitute self-determination are inherently social. This holds both for the social support to the capacity for reflecting on needs, desires, and possibilities, and for the social practices and organization that make some avenues of self-determination possible to some people, and close off others (Donchin 2000, 239).

Impairment both enriches and complicates our thinking about autonomy and agency. First, disability is generally characterized by deviation from the norm in terms of the disabled person's "interconnections with, and interdependencies upon, the body, others, and the structures of the world" (Ells 2001, 600). I want to stress again that this does *not* mean that disabled people are somehow connected with and dependent on the body and the social world, while nondisabled people are not. If we acknowledge that *everyone* is embodied, then we must also acknowledge that everyone experiences her life through the capacities and limits of the body. Equally, if we recognize that *everyone* is involved in a social fabric of dependencies and supports, the details of which vary from person to person, then everyone experiences her subjectivity through the constraints and opportunities offered by the social network. Embodiment and interdependence are realities for everyone, all the time. In a relational view of autonomy, self-determination can never be entirely down to the self because it is constituted in relationship (negotiation, compromise) with others. Under conditions of impairment, however, these universal features are experienced in unfamiliar ways, and they suddenly become more obvious.

This is an area of disability discourse where it really is necessary to think separately about physical and mental impairment. When there is cognitive limitation, or people are affected by mental illness, their capacity for making certain decisions or taking certain actions is often affected. (Even so, they still experience preferences and wishes, although someone else might have to enact them, and identifying these preferences and wishes may take effort and patience.) In the kinds of physical impairments I have mostly been considering, though, there should be no doubt that the cognitive and affective competences needed for self-determination remain intact. The disabled person will be perfectly clear about what is going on and what she wants, but she may be less able to act on her decisions. In these circumstances "the challenge for those with disability is to retain, regain, or re-figure substantial autonomy despite autonomy loss" (Ells 2001, 606), whether the loss is a direct effect of the impairment, or a consequence of the social and attitudinal barriers that prevent a person from exerting control.

One of the problems here is that when autonomy and disability are considered together, the terms of the bioethical conversation have a tendency to slip from talking about *autonomy* to evaluating relative *independence* in conditions with and without impairment. "Autonomy," if understood as the capacity to self-determine, is not synonymous with what people commonly mean by "independence." Caroline Ells points out that people who are ill or have impairments rarely use the term "autonomy," "which suggests that autonomy, at least as it is currently conceived, may not speak to their experience or needs" (599).[6] Solveig Magnus Reindal claims that disabled people are more likely to define *independence* as the "ability to be in control of and make decisions about one's life" (1999, 353), a definition that comes closer to the philosophical meaning of personal autonomy. The problem is that nondisabled people tend not to conceive of independence like this, but as something more like the ability to carry out life functions by oneself, without the help of anyone else. Trivially, people with various kinds of impairment often need forms of help that others do not. A person with a severe mobility impairment needs someone to assist her with washing, dressing, eating, and toileting. A less severely impaired person might need an assistance dog to retrieve objects from the floor. Someone with a hearing impairment may need a sign interpreter or subtitling to understand a spoken lecture. People without those impairments can wash, dress, pick up the fallen keys, and listen to the lecture independent of those kinds of help. By the criterion of "ability to perform functions by oneself," people without impairments are plainly more independent, while disabled people are generally less independent. If we then run independence into the capacity for self-determination too readily, it would be easy to conclude that disabled people are compromised in their autonomy as well.

The repercussions of the confusion of ideas around autonomy, independence, self-determination, and personhood are illustrated in the affective responses to the presumed loss or reduction of physical independence. To do justice to this issue needs more space than I have here, but it is widely recognized that contemporary Western societies respond badly to reduced independence. Loss of independence is (quite reasonably) associated with aging, which explains some of the response, but it is also accompanied by levels of fear and disgust that betray a less rational, infantile fear of the dissolution of interpersonal boundaries. Hence the need to deny or cover up dependence has enormous force. But it comes at a heavy price. As Susan Wendell says, "Some people will expend tremendous energy being 'independent' in ways that might be considered trivial in a culture less insistent on certain forms of self-reliance. . . . That energy [could be used] for more satisfying activities" (Wendell 1996, 147–48).

Permitted and Disallowed Dependencies

Recognizing asymmetric dependencies as ubiquitous is the starting point for a model in which societies are constituted by dependencies and responses to dependency. In any kind of social grouping some people need to call on others to do things they themselves can't in order simply to survive, let alone flourish. In more complex societies, the inability to live in absolute self-sufficiency arises for all sorts of biological, psychological, and social reasons: being young, old, or pregnant, smaller or taller than the norm, afraid of spiders, clueless about dressmaking, or not having time to grow one's own food. If everyone makes use of others in this way, it is clearly not the case that some people are dependent and others independent, but rather that some dependencies are permitted and other, disallowed ones are marked out as anomalous.⁷ What I call permitted dependencies are generally not seen as dependencies at all but as services that people are simply entitled to because they are "citizens who fit the social paradigms, who by definition are not considered dependent" (Wendell 1996, 40–41).

A feminist critique points out not only the ubiquity of permitted dependencies, but also that they are not natural phenomena. Permitted and disallowed dependencies are the result of social and political arrangements that could be arranged otherwise. It is worth pondering why, for example, a dependency on hearing aid batteries or a powered wheelchair is a "special need" when a dependency on electric light to see by is not. The usual answer to this is the quantitative one that only a small number of us use hearing aids or electric wheelchairs, but most people in Western societies use electricity, so it is normal to expect it to be provided.⁸ But this statement naturalizes something that is more contingent. There are parts of the world in which needing electric light to read by at night would be just as statistically anomalous as needing hearing aid batteries. And what about the provision of wireless Internet access, or power sockets on trains for commuters to plug in their laptops? Why a rail company will offer power points for laptops and razors, but not install visual as well as aural announcements, is a complicated question to do with choices about normality, fashion, markets, and communications. Here, I want only to highlight that the line between an entitlement (even when charged for) and a special need runs along a contour that has been selected, and which shifts with social changes and technological innovation. Once it is understood to be a line drawn by the accretion of unexamined social, political, and aesthetic decisions, however, the categories created by the line are denaturalized. By this I don't mean that there *is* no demarcation between special need and normal entitlement, or that there *should* never be one, but rather that choices have been made that also configure our moral stance toward impairment.

The discussion of dependencies in the feminist ethical literature is often conducted solely in terms of care ethics, and this has had an unfortunate effect on theorizing the relationship between impairment and dependency. First, it has alienated those disabled people, especially disability activists, who consider that the highest priority on the disability agenda is to ensure access to full civil and social participation. Many disability activists focus exclusively on the removal of the environmental and attitudinal barriers that prevent disabled people from entering the social worlds to which nondisabled people have readier access. According to the strong social model, once that access has been gained, disabled people will no longer need special allowance to be made, because they would then be able to support themselves and otherwise live just like any nondisabled person. Criticisms of this model were detailed earlier and will not be repeated here. But it is easy to see why from this perspective, care ethics' apparent veneration of carers presents a dangerously unbalanced view of disabled people. Some disability theorists hold that being the object of care necessarily undermines claims to equality (Silvers 1995). Activists sometimes accuse parents and professional carers of using care to justify an illegitimate level of control over disabled people's lives. Moreover, disability activists are sometimes critical of the place that the abstract ideal of care has taken in the cultural imagination of disability, arguing that paternalism or hostility is often disguised as care, for example in the often involuntary institutionalization of disabled children and adults in the nineteenth and twentieth centuries, or the enforced oralism of most twentieth-century education of hearing-impaired children.

Parents and other carers of disabled people, for their part, have countered that there are types and degrees of impairment that mean that some disabled people will never be able to participate fully in social life, however good their access to it is. Those with extensive impairments will always need some forms of physical assistance provided by their families or paid carers; severe cognitive impairments and some levels of multiple impairment inevitably reduce a person's capacity to live independently, as independence is commonly understood. For parents and carers, the chief concerns may not be discriminatory employment practices or lack of accessible toilets, but whether they will be able to provide lifelong care for the disabled member of their family without destroying their own lives and health in the process. From *this* perspective, unjust discrimination against disabled people is instantiated by inadequate or absent state support for carers, or employment cultures that make it impossible to work part-time or flexibly in order to support disabled dependents.

Setting up the "full social participation" and the "adequate social support" agendas as a polar opposition between disabled people themselves and (paternalistic) carers has led to the theoretical resources provided by the feminist ethic of care being as neglected in disability studies as in bioethics. Although early work in care ethics (Gilligan 1982; Noddings 1984; Tronto 1993) focused on the gendered nature of distinct modes of moral discourse, more recently there has been a move toward recognizing multiple moral "voices," not necessarily separated along the axis of gender, that are more or less dominant according to context and the type of ethical work being done (Hekman 1995). The concept of care in ethics is not solely about some people (usually, but not always, women) doing the physical work of looking after the body needs of dependent others, although this aspect has received the most attention in medical and, particularly, nursing ethics. The approach of care ethics is rather to foreground individual and community connections with others, with an emphasis on acknowledging dependencies and interdependencies as a basis for moral response. To imagine people as not fully autonomous, but always in a condition of interdependence, as Joan Tronto puts it, "allows us to understand both autonomous and involved elements of human life" (1993, 162).

Care ethics pays closest attention to the contextual detail of relational bonds of affect and obligation between intimates. Even its proponents agree there are theoretical difficulties in scaling up a morality that is based around so-called caring relationships for application to the moral struggles of larger social units, where personal connections are often nonexistent or obscured. Arguably, what the ethic of care has most to offer at a social and policy level is its capacity to shift the epistemic frame within which we acknowledge certain dependencies as normal but identify others as "special." Despite its usual focus on the small-scale, care ethics' alertness to the characteristics of nonreciprocal relationships also gives fresh insight into the structure of larger-scale nonreciprocal dependencies and, distinctively, into the affective, nonrational reactions behind the social responses to permitted and disallowed dependence.

Reimagining Self-Determination

In the lives of disabled people whose capacity for self-determination, as measured by conventional standards, is reduced, the experience of impairment often demands a reimagining of what being in control or independent can mean. Autonomy and related capacities can be constituted in forms that we fail to recognize as such. In the study I have already described in which people with candidate conditions for somatic gene therapy were asked about its ethics, clinicians and patients differed markedly in the features they identified as giving them more control over their lives (Scully et al. 2004). Clinicians saw the independence of patients increasing in direct proportion to a reduction in their vulnerability to disease symptoms. Yet our participants with cystic fibrosis, multiple sclerosis, or familial cancer often located "control" elsewhere than in symptom reduction per se. They also tended to express it in terms of relationship rather than symptoms or functionality. For example, some said that being able to show care for their children by collecting them from school was most important to them. Their fear was that an experimental treatment, which they imagined would demand more time in the clinic, would reduce rather than increase their autonomy, whatever it did for their symptoms. Other participants were worried that, even if the treatment worked well, they would become in some way "dependent" on the therapy, and that in itself would harm their sense of being in control of their lives.

Jonathan Cole has studied the lives of men paralyzed by spinal cord injury (Cole 2004). One of the tetraplegic men he interviewed says, "I appreciate being completely in control of my own circumstances." For him, however, this means not that he necessarily acts independently, but that he employs someone as an assistant, to do "the things I can't do for myself in day to day living." He does not consider this assistant as a carer, but as a medium through which he exerts his control over his environment (72). Similarly, Cole describes an interviewee, Stephen, gaining "a sense of agency and ownership of action for himself" in the task of washing up, by asking his personal assistant to do it. Controversially—and this is an area that cries out for further ethical and sociological study—Cole argues that a good PA can, temporarily and voluntarily, relinquish part of his or her own agency and transfer it to the tetraplegic person through the agreement between them that the tetraplegic employer can order actions when and exactly how she wants. Cole takes up Merleau-Ponty's account of embodiment and paraphrasing and extends it to the PA: "Consciousness can be a being-toward-the-thing through the intermediary of my body and that of my PA. . . . My body and that of my PA are the general media for having a world" (289).

These examples come from the lives of people who have lost the ability to exercise some taken-for-granted kinds of control, and for whom the difference before and after the loss is most marked. I've noted before that there is less empirical work and fewer subjective accounts of the lifelong experience of marked phenotypic anomaly, that is, people for whom bodily difference is their normality. In practice it is methodologically harder to discern subtle perceptual and cognitive differences that might result from altered embodiment when that "alteration" is a person's norm. Still, it is possible to indicate some promising avenues. In chapter 5 we saw that although cognitive science has so far concentrated on the standard body form, the embodied mind model suggests that alterations in phenotype might influence higher-order cognitive functions, including abstract conceptualization. If we are willing to allow this, we might also be willing to consider the extent to which habitual and repeated interaction with prostheses or human or animal assistants are incorporated into the body schema, becoming phenomenologically part of the body's cognitive and agential capacities. Or we might want to take the concept of relational autonomy and examine the role of communities like the Deaf world, groupings around specific impairments, or the disability community as a whole in the production of personal autonomy and identity. Disability studies has done so to an extent, and feminist ethics' long and thorough engagement with issues of identity politics has prepared some of the ground here. By contrast, mainstream bioethics has yet to attempt a proper account of the ethical implications of identity and identity politics.

Ideas like these merit careful investigation because interactions between assistance (human or mechanical) and the disabled person will not *automatically* enhance the autonomy of the latter: that will depend on whose choice the interaction is, and how it is done. Some people do well with a prosthetic limb. They find that it improves the range of functions they can perform and they may incorporate it into their body schemas. But for others, as the stories of Diane DeVries (Frank 2000) and Alison Lapper (2005) show, prostheses are imposed on them as a result of nondisabled people defining what independence should look like, and expecting phenotypically variant people to go along with it. The result will be unethical if, for example, a nondisabled ideal of independence is used to set the parameters for provision of supports and services, or if disabled people are made to feel inadequate, or are deprived of a habitus where they feel at home, because they fail to live up to someone else's functional ideal.

Social-relational models argue that the significantly restricted capacity for self-determination that disabled people may experience does not result solely from the impairment itself, but through constraints operating at the interface between the body and social world. The *bad thing* of disability is a consequence of interactions that frustrate the possibilities of self-determination a disabled person would otherwise have. The moral fault here does not lie with oppressive societies *tout court*, as the strong social model would say, but in the fact that some possibilities for self-determination are contingently frustrated through attitudes and social organizations that are, in practice, open to change. If autonomy is an achievement of embodied social interaction rather than a property a person stably and constantly *has* (Ells 2001), then the ethical requirement to respect autonomy asks for something rather more substantial than not interfering with a patient's decisions about treatment options. Bioethics would need to examine in ethical terms the barriers that get in the way of a disabled person's exercising self-determination through interconnection with others, as much as the better-recognized problems of barriers to access. A full account of such barriers would implicate economic, environmental, social, cultural, and psychological forces of the kind that do not generally feature in mainstream moral philosophy's discourse on autonomy.

THE BODY IN MORAL UNDERSTANDING

Just as bioethics has recently undergone an empirical turn, other disciplines have taken what we might call a body swerve. Sociology, history, and cultural studies are among the areas with a growing literature theorizing the body, while feminist theory has not surprisingly given closest attention to gendered bodily difference (Diprose 1994; Grosz 1994, 1995; Weiss 1999; Bordo 2004). As Shakespeare and Watson (1996) point out, however, from the viewpoint of disability, the sociological engagement with the body was, until recently, inadequate. The sociology of the body focuses on "exotic" phenomena such as transgressive sexual identities, body manipulation, and the body as a consumer commodity or a discursive construct. It has shown much less interest in lived experience, including the lived experience of disability and impairment where a physically determinist line is generally preferred. At the same time, some of the recent feminist work on the body has—rightly, in my view—been accused of having an obsession (Garland-Thomson 2002, 9) with fantastic, "monstrous" bodies, while being seemingly oblivious to the many embodiments that already transgress somatic norms (Haraway 1991, 1997; Braidotti 1994, 2002). Thus this work reveals itself to be interested in bodily variation, but only limited types of variant and only, it seems, on its own terms.

Yet to many scholars, returning the body to academic inquiry smacks dangerously of attempts to tie subjectivities down to an unchanging, biologically determined essence. This is what makes body theory problematic for feminist, race, or gay/lesbian/transgender theory. There are long-standing tensions between the socially and politically progressive projects in which these theories are rooted, and the apparent conservatism of biological or indeed any other form of essentialism. Focusing on the material body, or so the argument goes, is bound to dilute the efficacy of any movement concerned with transforming the social identities associated with certain embodiments. This anxiety was challenged by Diane Fuss some years ago; she pointed out the ease with which it is taken for granted that "nature and fixity go together (naturally) just as sociality and change go together (naturally) . . . it may be time to ask whether essences can change and whether constructions can be normative" (Fuss 1989, 6). For disability theory, anxiety about body essentialism is linked to the fear of separating off disabled people into the category marked "irrevocably different," thus rolling back all the effort of the past thirty years to move disabled people out of the marginal social spaces into which they are often pushed. The progressive hope of the disability movement is to reconfigure disabled people as "just people" with moral and legal rights to the same civil goods that nondisabled people enjoy. For its part, disability studies aims to theorize disability and impairment without undoing the social and political advances that have already been achieved. But to some critics, the reemergence of the body in disability discourse threatens to do exactly that.

Feminism's existing work on the body and identity can inform disability bioethics' own engagement with the body. What may be especially valuable is feminism's theoretical capacity to admit "disability" (like "women") as a discursive category, while at the same time not losing a grip on the bodily particularities that make it possible to construct this particular discursive category in the first place. Feminist theory therefore offers disability bioethics the resources for thinking about embodied being in ways that recognize the "debt" that identity owes to the body (Bell 1999, 132), while leaving open the conceptual space to examine how phenotypically variant bodies are culturally identified. It is quite a trick, to be able to notice how "our ideas and attitudes seep into the functioning of the body itself, making up the realm of its possibilities or impossibilities" (Grosz 1994, 190), and to do this without forgetting that there *really are* possibilities and impossibilities that cannot be dismissed as the effects of discourse. Feminist theory attempts to give accounts of the body that resist the temptation to pin it down as *either* biological *or* social, but allow it to be simultaneously composed of limiting parameters *and* sites open to manipulation and change.

I haven't said much about bioethics in this section, largely because so far the discipline has shown an almost total lack of interest in embodiment. Until recently it could be said in bioethics' defense that the analyses needed to do so were undeveloped. That position is rapidly becoming less convincing as the theoretical and methodological tools offered by contemporary science and philosophy become more sophisticated. Given the basic subject matter of bioethics, its neglect of the body is extraordinary. And just as bioethical discourse is enriched by the inclusion of feminism's insights into gendered bodies, it would also profit from the insights into anomalous or impaired bodies that disability theory offers. Disability theory's account of the body is distinguished by two things: that it has to deal with the fact that impairment is a good deal more diverse than other categories of embodiment, like gender or race; and that impairment is associated with degrees of potential intrinsic disadvantage in ways that other characteristics are not. Gendered embodiment, for example, goes along with certain advantages and disadvantages that are wholly cultural. The *bad thing* about being a woman, if we can put it like that, is derivative on the specifics of female biology. If there is a disadvantage to female embodiment, it comes from living in social arrangements that ensure that bodies biologically defined as female are socially inferior, exploited, physically abused, and so on. These disadvantages are cultural because they could be, and in some times and places are, otherwise. Similar points can be made about raced embodiment. I don't think this is always the case with disability, and therein lies the prime difficulty for both disability theory and bioethics. I consider this further in the next section.

ONTOLOGICAL MEANINGS OF IMPAIRMENT

Impairment and disability present bioethics with tricky questions. Usually the ethical difficulties in disability are not black-or-white dilemmas that involve one moral stance facing down another. More commonly, the issues are rather diffuse, needing careful description and examination, and involving differences in interpretation and priorities rather than stark confrontations. Nevertheless, behind all ethical work on disability lies the single intractable question that impairment presents to bioethicists and everyone else: What is its ontological meaning? What ought we to think about disability? Is phenotypic variation beyond a certain point inherently undesirable, something that we ought always to prevent or remove if we can? Or does phenotypic variation bring enough (or any) benefits to our lives, individually and socially, that a positive response to it is feasible?

Some bioethicists will be unconvinced that bioethics needs to work with the question of impairment in any way differently than it has done before. They may hold that genetic and other biomedical technologies will one day be able to ensure that phenotypic variation is minimized or eliminated altogether.[9] If so, then there is no need to expand bioethics' understanding of what it is like to live with impairment, since quite soon it will not be a pressing ethical issue. I think this position is mistaken, for two reasons. One is that it rests on the hope that all impairments can be prevented by prenatal or preimplantation diagnoses coupled to appropriate interventions. Of course a minority of impairments are genetically determined, while many more are influenced to some degree by genotype. Still, quantitatively the most significant causes of impairment are accidents, war, illness, or aging, areas of life where genetic diagnosis has less impact. It may be countered that there could turn out to be strong genetic determinants of aging and of vulnerabilities to infection or even susceptibility to trauma, and that these will eventually be unraveled so that genetic diagnosis would help shield populations from them. The available scientific evidence suggests that this is unlikely to happen in the near future, and even less likely—given political and economic realities—to be made available everywhere. So, even if *known* genetically determined conditions could be eradicated from affluent, technologically developed societies, people would continue to be disabled in those societies for nongenetic reasons, and elsewhere in the world for all reasons.

The second objection cuts closer to the troubled heart of bioethics' relationship with impairment. Expecting the problem of disability to be solved by preventing impairment appearing in the first place assumes that phenotypic variation is, as a rule, unwanted. I've been indicating that the reality is much more complicated (and more interesting) than that. It is true that the consequences of extensive phenotypic variation are often profoundly disadvantageous. There are impairments which are lethal in infancy, cause unbearable physical pain, or in other ways seem incompatible with a life anyone would choose to live. We can acknowledge all that and still not reject the intuition of many disabled and nondisabled people that eradicating all disadvantageous phenotypic variation would entail losses as well as gains.

In many years of following conversations about disability between disability theorists and (usually nondisabled) bioethicists, I've noted how often the "magic pill" hypothetical is presented as a kind of trump card. In the
magic pill hypothetical the disabled person is asked whether, if a magic pill
were available that would restore her sight or mobility or hearing and so on,
immediately and painlessly and cheaply, would she take it? This is a
philosopher's thought experiment that actually contains at least three different questions. First is the overt (1) wouldn't *you* prefer to be unimpaired?
Many disabled people will happily answer "yes," and if they do that's the
end of it. But when the response is (as it can be) "no" or "I'm not sure,"
what usually happens is that the questioner won't leave it there, and will
press on in a way that reveals the hidden second and third questions which
the first has failed to answer: (2) however *you* feel about it, wouldn't it be
better if impairment in general could be prevented or completely repaired?
and (3) ultimately, wouldn't it be better if phenotypic variation as a rule
could be prevented?

It seems to me that we cannot yet answer questions two and three. Partly,
this is because we haven't previously had to think about effective prevention or repair as practical possibilities, and so we have yet to give them focused consideration. But it is also partly because our social organizations
are currently still so hostile toward nonstandard embodiments. If disability
is a phenomenon generated at the interfaces of the biological body with the
material, social, and psychic worlds, as the social-relational models suggest,
then the desirability versus disadvantage of variation must also be tracked
along these interfaces. And if the biological versus cultural/social/material
contributions to disability cannot be readily disentangled from each other,
and if none of the contributing factors is entirely malleable or entirely fixed,
then for quite a lot of phenotypic variation the outcome (the lived reality)
will be sensitive to manipulation of *any* of the biological, cultural, social, or
material inputs.

Many disability theorists (but not all) will agree with me that in many
(but not all) cases, phenotypic variation *is* impairment. In these cases there
are elements of intrinsic disadvantage that cannot be avoided or eradicated
by social restructuring or cultural change. Sometimes, indeed, the variation
is so profoundly damaging and painful that most people would not hesi-
tate to say it justifies prenatal or preconception intervention to prevent the
birth of people who would experience it. However, in many other cases, a
larger part of the disadvantage is constituted by social responses to phenotypic anomaly. Since no society I can think of has entirely eliminated the
social or cultural contributions to disablement, the magnitude of the intrinsic disadvantage is only really clear when it is so overwhelming that it
renders the other contributions trivial. For many phenotypic variations, it is
not yet possible to assess how much intrinsic disadvantage would be left

over if social responses were different. Clearly there are also other questions to resolve, such as how to measure the different contributing factors, and then how to decide which factor or factors make the larger contribution or are more readily modifiable. But a better grasp of what the experience is like, and what it *can* be like under changed conditions, would at least give firmer grounds on which to base bioethical judgments about intrinsic and modifiable disadvantage.

Questions two and three also screen an array of other issues about costs and benefits. The magic pill hypothetical is meaningless because it postulates that the biotechnologies involved come at no economic or other cost. In the real world, biomedical research and healthcare provision use financial resources and take up researchers' and developers' time. Even magic pills cost money. Still, before rushing to conclude that the economic, political, or personal cost of magic pills is too high, we should not forget that social or political rearrangements aiming to reduce the marginalization of disabled people do not take place in a vacuum either. They too will have economic and other impacts. The bioethical discussion of PND, PGD, surgical interventions for disabled people, and so on needs not only to take these economic features into account as best it can; it also needs to consider how and why issues around phenotypic abnormality have been presented as bioethical rather than economic or policy topics (Haimes 2002, Hedgecoe 2004). Questions two and three can be rephrased as: would it be worth preventing/repairing impairment in general, or only prenatally, if it costs x and has y efficacy? To address these questions, a critical disability bioethics will draw on empirical and subjective evidence of the experience of disability to inform its reasoning about relative costs, benefits, and impacts. It needs to consider too the *nature* of the costs and impacts that are routinely taken into ethical account. Becoming more familiar with others' lived experience of disability may indicate that there are other terms of reference (emotional, aesthetic, social, or spiritual ones) that are relevant to an issue like impairment.

I want to make it quite clear that disability bioethics would not inevitably conclude (for example) that selecting against certain kinds of impairment, where we can, is morally unacceptable. A properly critical and self-critical disability bioethics would be just as wary of claims that societies are enriched by the presence of impairment, that suffering improves human character, or that the vulnerabilities of some people call forth sterling qualities of compassion out of others as it would be of overheated biomedical hype. All such claims need to be examined very closely to see who is making them, on what authority, and what sorts of benefits they confer and to whom. Some people, both disabled and nondisabled, feel that all forms of disadvantaging phenotypic variation ought to be prevented if possible. Other people, both disabled and nondisabled, claim that all forms of phenotypic diversity should be unreservedly welcomed and celebrated. Such claims effectively erase the enriching along with the frustrating and distressing aspects of disabled people's experience. They become less convincing as the full range of that experience is recognized.

ETHICS OF RECOGNITION

Recognition is a key theme for disability bioethics. Recognition can be withheld from other people by all sorts of means: ignoring their existence entirely, relying on stereotypes about them, taking them as unfathomably other (so it is not worth trying to understand them), or alternatively assuming that we and they are the same (so there is no need to try because we already understand them), or thinking we can nevertheless put ourselves into their shoes. By contrast, the alternative I've outlined is all about recognizing others' experience, and recognizing the partial nature of our own knowledge. It suggests a need to acquire as much empirical and other information about impairment as possible, while at the same time acknowledging that such data do not enable nondisabled observers to occupy the same epistemic or moral space around impairment. Nor does recognizing another's subjectivity require us to agree that her beliefs and perceptions are right, or accept her moral understandings as necessarily good or authoritative, although the knowledge we gain might result in our coming to a different conclusion than before.

But whatever the effect on individual judgments, the *decision* to give serious attention to the embodied experiences of impairment is an ethical act in itself. It is a moral choice to respect (though not uncritically) a disabled person's accounting of her own life. Identity formation is a social process: an individual's selfhood consolidates around how she is regarded by others. As a result, her sense of self is generated not only from her own experience of her embodiment, but also from her experience of how others respond to it. Although I can't offer more solid evidence than personal knowledge and the stories of other disabled people, it does seem that a major element in the overall quality of life of many phenotypically variant people is whether they are constantly regarded as anomalous by their community or, conversely, are accepted as part of that community's normality. Some disabled people will have spaces where they are acknowledged as normal (perhaps among people who know them very well, within the Deaf community, or, for some, the disability activist world). But for many others with bodies that are noticeably phenotypically variant, such spaces are rare or absent. The larger social world withholds recognition of the aspects of their experience that are seen as odd, best ignored, or to be excused.

Bioethicists, then, have an ethical requirement to show respect for disabled others through epistemic openness to the empirical and subjective facts of their lives. In case I appear to be making disproportionate demands of bioethicists here, this ethical responsibility is placed on others, too, disability scholars included. The disability movement has sometimes shown its own kind of inability to deal with the full range of impairment experiences, denying unwanted aspects such as weakness, pain, vulnerability, premature death, physical limitation, and frustration, which do not fit comfortably with the positive political image of what Cheryl Marie Wade called "the able-disabled" (1994, 35, cited in Wendell 1996, 146). When that happens, disability theory withholds moral recognition from (the wrong kinds of) disabled people as effectively as anyone who actively stereotypes them or denies that some kinds of disability identity exist.

As I write this in the summer of 2007, I have been deaf for almost thirty-six years. In all that time, not one hearing person has ever asked me the question, "What is like to hear as you do?" What they ask is, "How much can you hear?" Over the years I've come to think that these two apparently similar questions have secondary meanings that are fundamentally quite different. The first question means: *tell me the truth of your experience.* The second means: *how do you measure up against my standard?* Of course, there is nothing wrong with asking that second question. It gets asked for legitimate, good reasons, for example when people want to know how to make practical arrangements to ensure that I can participate on equal terms. Nevertheless, it continues to intrigue me, and it accords with the accounts by disabled writers such as Wendell, Johnson, and Hockenberry that nondisabled people seem unable to imagine there could be illuminating or even enjoyable aspects to phenotypic variation, or that there are aspects to the experience the nondisabled majority might just find worth knowing about. When John Hockenberry asks, "What would a world look like in which people would dare to wish to know what it is like not to walk?" (Hockenberry 1995, 214), he's not claiming that everyone should want *not* to be able to walk, but that the resounding lack of curiosity about what it is like to live from a wheelchair[10] is indicative of a peculiarly rigid stance toward the presence of varied embodiment.

So where do we go from here? I have argued that disability is best served by a bioethics that is critical, self-critical, and rooted in empirical and phenomenological or existential-phenomenological knowledge of impairment. What I described as a mainstream ethics of disability approach to questions of impairment, primarily concerned with regulating selective or therapeutic technologies, can become more critical and self-critical, but it also needs to be complemented by a parallel disability bioethics mode of thought. In analogy to feminist bioethics, disability bioethics starts its reflections from the diversity of experiences of impairment, drawing on these epistemic resources as well as on the skeptical sociopolitical analytic tools of feminist and disability theorists. Although the two approaches run in parallel, it is inevitable (and desirable) that disability bioethics will both feed into and be fed by the more mainstream bioethics of disability.

Developing a disability bioethics does a good deal more than enlarge the cultural catalog entitled *weird stuff about other people*. For one thing, it starts to uncover the implicit background of beliefs about normality on which moral philosophers and bioethicists base their normative statements about impairment and other kinds of perceived deviance. Disability bioethics helps philosophy become attuned to the practices of representation and self-representation of the moral agents with which it is concerned; this is important, because the finding that a social identity (of a disabled person in this case) is vulnerable to systematic misrepresentation has repercussions for the reliability of the epistemic resources that serve philosophical thinking as a whole. The job of bioethics would then have to include close examination of the representations, narratives, and cultural practices that generate those resources and encourage the provision of better ones.

At points along the way I have indicated that a critical examination of bioethics' epistemic resources will inevitably raise additional questions about how, exactly, people with impairments are best enabled to contribute constructively to bioethical debates. There is already growing interest in public engagement and consultation processes around biomedicine, drawing on theoretical sources running from Habermasian discourse ethics to Rawlsian reflective equilibrium. Although enhancing lay involvement is not a universal panacea for all bioethics' epistemological limits (see Ashcroft [2003] for a further discussion of this), most bioethicists would probably consider it a step in the right direction.[11] So far, however, the bioethical discussion here has concentrated on models of practice and process that best facilitate public involvement in general (see, for example, Banks et al. 2006). Little or no detailed thought has been given to the additional barriers to participation faced by disabled people—most obviously barriers of mobility and communication, but also the less familiar ones of vocabulary, history, financial resources, time, or energy.

The expansion of bioethical attention to these considerations of power and process, to the mundane, embodied features of situations and agents, underlines the family resemblance between disability bioethics and feminist bioethics. Like feminist bioethics, disability bioethics is not about solving the problem of an anomaly, but about understanding specific ways of being in the world, and doing so in the hope that such understanding will help to improve the lives of disabled people. The effort of extending, clarifying, and challenging bioethical reflection on disability is not *just* about doing better philosophy or better disability studies. It is part of a moral commitment to asking the right questions of impairment and normality as the basis for producing what we hope are the right answers.

NOTES

1. The title paraphrases Dennis Potter's *The Singing Detective* (BBC TV 1986), whose main character says: "All clues and no solutions. That's how things really are. Plenty of clues; no solutions."

2. This is not a special attack on bioethicists. As disabled people are a minority in Western societies, and because there is considerable social pressure not to be identified as impaired, *most* people lack the kind of personal experience or close contact I refer to here.

3. An example of a feminist critique of the place of autonomy in medical ethics can be found in Dodds (2000).

4. I don't mean by this that there is something intrinsically wrong with patients' having freedom of choice, of course, only that this is an oversimplification of even Beauchamp and Childress' discussion of autonomy, and an emaciated version of the concept of autonomy in moral philosophy.

5. There is more than one theory of autonomy in contemporary "mainstream" philosophy, and more than one kind of feminist or communitarian philosophical critique; the sketch I have given here for the sake of conciseness does not do justice to either the mainstream or the critical arguments. For a comprehensive overview and more detailed analysis, see the collected essays in Mackenzie and Stoljar (2000).

6. It is doubtful, though, whether in fact many nonphilosophers, disabled or not, use the term "autonomy" much either.

7. See also the discussions in Wendell (1996) and in Morris (1991).

8. I mean provided as a product to be bought. This is not an argument about which supports should be provided free of charge, but about which needs are defined as normal.

9. I am not entering into the debate about enhancement and improvement technologies, since some different questions arise there; Christoph Rehmann-Sutter and I have argued that disability destabilizes the distinction between therapy and enhancement. See Scully and Rehmann-Sutter (2001).

10. Waist-high in the world, as Nancy Mairs (1996) puts it.

11. Some have expressed more reservation about the uses to which public opinion is put: see Harris (2005).

References

Abberley, P. 1987. "The concept of oppression and the development of a social theory of disability." *Disability, Handicap and Society* 2:5–21.

Ahmad, W. I. U. 2000. *Ethnicity, Disability and Chronic Illness*. Buckingham: Open University Press.

Albrecht, G. L., and P. J. Devliger. 1999. "The disability paradox: High quality of life against all odds." *Social Science & Medicine* 48:977–88.

Alford, C. F. 1991. *The Self in Social Theory: A Psychoanalytic Account of Its Construction in Plato, Hobbes, Locke, Rawls, and Rousseau*. New Haven, Conn.: Yale University Press.

Amundsen, R. 2005. "Disability, ideology, and quality of life: a bias in biomedical ethics." In Wasserman et al., pp. 101–24.

Anspach, R. R. 1993. *Deciding Who Lives: Fateful Choices in the Intensive-Care Nursery*. Berkeley: University of California Press.

Anstey, K. W. 2002. "Are attempts to have impaired children justifiable?" *Journal of Medical Ethics* 28:286–88.

Appiah, K. A. 1994. "Identity, authenticity, survival: Multicultural societies and social reproduction." In *Multiculturalism*, ed. A. Gutmann, pp. 149–64. Princeton, N.J.: Princeton University Press.

———. 2004. *The Ethics of Identity*. Princeton, N.J.: Princeton University Press.

Asch, A., and D. Wasserman. 2005. "What is the sin in synecdoche? Prenatal testing and the parent-child relationship." In Wasserman et al., pp. 172–216.

Ashcroft, R. E. 2003. "Constructing empirical bioethics: Foucauldian reflections on the empirical turn in bioethics research." *Health Care Analysis* 11:3–13.

———. 2005. "Power, corruption and lies: Ethics and power." In *Case Analysis in Clinical Ethics*, ed. R. Ashcroft, A. Lucassen, M. Parker, M. Verkerk, and G. Widdershoven, pp. 77–94. Cambridge: Cambridge University Press.

Baier, A. 1985. *Postures of the Mind: Essays on Mind and Morals*. London: Methuen.

Banks, S., J. L. Scully, and T. Shakespeare. 2006. "Ordinary ethics: Lay people's deliberations on social sex selection." *New Genetics and Society* 25:289–303.

Barnes, C. 1998. "The social model of disability: A sociological phenomenon ignored by sociologists?" In Shakespeare, pp. 65–78.

Barnes, C., G. Mercer, and T. Shakespeare. 1999. *Exploring Disability: A Sociological Introduction*. Cambridge: Polity Press.

Bartky, S. L. 1990. *Femininity and Domination: Studies in the Phenomenology of Oppression*. London: Taylor & Francis.

———. 2002. *Sympathy and Solidarity*. Lanham, Md.: Rowman & Littlefield.

Baruch, S., D. Kaufman, and K. Hudson. 2008. "Genetic testing of embryos: Practices and perspectives of U.S. IVF clinics." *Fertility and Sterility* 89:1053–8.

Beauchamp, T., and J. Childress. 2001. *Principles of Biomedical Ethics*. 5th ed. Oxford: Oxford University Press.

Becker, G. 2000. *The Elusive Embryo: How Men and Women Approach New Reproductive Technologies*. Berkeley: University of California Press.

Bell, V. 1999. *Feminist Imagination: Genealogies in Feminist Theory*. London: Sage.

Benhabib, S. 2002. *The Claims of Culture: Equality and Diversity in the Global Era*. Princeton, N.J.: Princeton University Press.

Berlucchi, G., and S. Aglioti. 1997. "The body in the brain: Neural bases of corporeal awareness." *Trends in Neurosciences* 20:560–64.

Bérubé, M. 1996. *Life as We Know It: A Father, a Family, and an Exceptional Child*. New York: Pantheon.

Boorse, C. 1977. "Health as a theoretical concept." *Philosophy of Science* 44:542–73.

Bordo, S. 1990. "Feminism, postmodernism, and gender-scepticism." In *Feminism/Postmodernism*, ed. L. J. Nicholson, pp. 133–56. London: Routledge.

———. 2004. *Unbearable Weight: Feminism, Western Culture and the Body*. Berkeley: University of California Press.

Borry, P., P. Schotsmans, and K. Dierickx. 2005. "The birth of the empirical turn in bioethics." *Bioethics* 19:49–71.

———. 2006. "Empirical research in bioethical journals: A quantitative analysis." *Journal of Medical Ethics* 32:240–45.

Borsay, A. 2005. *Disability and Social Policy in Britain since 1750: A History of Exclusion*. Basingstoke, UK: Palgrave.

Bourdieu, P. 1990. *In Other Words: Essays towards a Reflexive Sociology*. Trans. M. Adamson. Stanford, Calif.: Stanford University Press.

———. 1993. *Sociology in Question*. Trans. R. Nice. London: Sage. [Orig. pub. as *Questions de Sociologie* by Éditions de Minuit, Paris, 1984.]

———. 2000. *Pascalian Meditations*. Cambridge: Polity Press.

Bourdieu, P., and T. Eagleton. 1992. "Doxa and common life," edited transcript of a discussion at the Institute of Contemporary Arts, London, May 15, 1991. *New Left Review* January–February:111–21.

Boyle, T. C. 2006. *Talk Talk*. New York: Viking.

Braddock, D. L., and S. L. Parish. 2001. "An institutional history of disability." In *The Disability Studies Handbook*, ed. A. Gary, K. Seelman, and M. Bury, pp. 11–60. London: Sage.

Braidotti, R. 1994. *Nomadic Subjects: Embodiment and Sexual Difference in Contemporary Feminist Theory.* New York: Columbia University Press.

———. 2002. *Metamorphoses: Towards a Materialist Theory of Becoming.* Cambridge: Polity Press.

Brody, B. 1993. "Assessing empirical research in bioethics." *Theoretical Medicine* 14:211–19.

Brown, W. 1993. "Wounded attachments." *Political Theory* 21:390–410.

Buchanan, A. 1996. "Choosing who will be disabled: Genetic intervention and the morality of inclusion." *Social Philosophy and Policy* 13:18–46.

Buchanan, A., D.W. Brock, N. Daniels, and D. Wikler. 2000. *From Chance to Choice: Genetics and Justice.* Cambridge: Cambridge University Press.

Bull, T. H. 1998. *On the Edge of Deaf Culture: Hearing Children/Deaf Parents.* Alexandria, Va.: Deaf Family Research Press.

Butler, G. E., and E. E. Beadle. 2007. "Manipulating growth and puberty in those with severe disability: When is it justified?" *Archives of Disease in Childhood* 92:567–68.

Butler, J. 1990. *Gender Trouble—Feminism and the Subversion of Identity.* New York: Routledge.

Calhoun, C. 1989. "Responsibility and Reproach." *Ethics* 99:389–406.

Campbell, J., and M. Oliver. 1996. *Disability Politics: Understanding Our Past, Changing Our Future.* London: Routledge.

Card, C. 2002. "Responsibility ethics, shared understandings, and moral communities." *Hypatia* 17:141–55.

Chase, B. W., T. A. Cornille, and R. W. English. 2000. "Life satisfaction among persons with spinal cord injuries." *Journal of Rehabilitation* 66:14–20.

Chorost, M. 2005. *Rebuilt: How Becoming Part Computer Made Me More Human.* New York: Houghton Mifflin.

Clare, E. 1999. *Exile and Pride: Disability, Queerness and Liberation.* Cambridge, Mass.: South End Press.

Code, L. 1991. *What Can She Know? Feminist Theory and the Construction of Knowledge.* Ithaca, N.Y.: Cornell University Press.

———. 2002. "Narratives of responsibility and agency: Reading Margaret Walker's *Moral Understandings.*" *Hypatia* 17:156–73.

Cole, J. 2004. *Still Lives: Narratives of Spinal Cord Injury.* Chester, N.J.: Bradford Books.

Corker, M. 1998a. "Derrida on disability—reconstructing the social model?" Unpublished conference paper, presented to Society of Disability Studies, Oakland, Calif.

———. 1998b. *Deaf and Disabled, or Deafness Disabled?* Buckingham: Open University Press.

———. 1999. "Differences, conflations and foundations: The limits to 'accurate' theoretical representation of disabled people's experience." *Disability and Society* 14:627–42.

———. 2002. "Deafness/disability—problematising notions of identity, culture and structure." In *Disability, Culture and Identity,* ed. S. Ridell and N. Watson, pp. 88–104. London: Pearson.

Couser, G. T. 1997. *Recovering Bodies: Illness, Disability and Life Writing.* Madison: University of Wisconsin Press.

Craig, A. D. 2002. "How do you feel? Interoception: The sense of the physiological condition of the body." *Nature Reviews Neuroscience* 3:655–66.

Crouch, R. A. 1997. "Letting the deaf be Deaf: Reconsidering the use of cochlear implants in prelingually deaf children." *Hastings Center Report* 4:14–21.

Crow, L. 1996. "Including all of our lives: Renewing the social model of disability." In *Encounters with Strangers: Feminism and Disability,* ed. J. Morris, pp. 206–22. London: Women's Press.

Cumberbatch, G., and R. Negrine. 1992. *Images of Disability on Television.* London: Routledge.

Cushman, L. A., and M. P. Dijkers. 1990. "Depressed mood in spinal cord injured persons: Staff perceptions and patient realities." *Archives of Physical Medicine and Rehabilitation* 71:191–96.

Danermark, B., and L. C. Gellerstedt. 2004. "Social justice: redistribution and recognition—a non-reductionist perspective on disability." *Disability and Society* 19:339–53.

Daniels, N. 1987. *Justice and Health Care.* In *Health Care Ethics: An Introduction,* ed. D. Van De Veer and T. Regan, pp. 290–325. Philadelphia: Temple University Press.

Darke, P. 1998. "Understanding cinematic representation of disability." In Shakespeare, pp. 181–197.

Darling, R. B. 2003. "Toward a model of changing disability identities: A proposed typology and research agenda." *Disability and Society* 18:881–95.

Davies, M., and T. Stone. 1995. *Mental Simulation.* Oxford: Blackwell.

Davis, D. 1997. "Genetic dilemmas and the child's right to an open future." *Hastings Center Report* 27:7–15.

———. 2001. *Genetic Dilemmas: Reproductive Technology, Parental Choices, and Children's Futures.* New York: Routledge.

De Preester, H. 2007. "The deep bodily origins of the subjective perspective: Models and their problems." *Consciousness and Cognition* 16:604–16.

DeVries, R. 2002. "How can we help? From 'sociology in' to 'sociology of' bioethics." *Journal of Law, Medicine & Ethics* 32:279–92.

DeVries, R., and J. Subedi, eds. 1998. *Bioethics and Society: Constructing the Ethical Enterprise.* N.J.: Prentice Hall.

DeVries, R., L. Turner, K. Orfali, C. Bosk, eds. 2007. *The View from Here: Bioethics and the Social Sciences.* Oxford: Wiley-Blackwell.

Diprose, R. 1994. *The Bodies of Women.* London: Routledge.

Dodds, S. 2000. "Choice and control in feminist bioethics." In Mackenzie and Stoljar, pp. 213–35.

Donchin, A. 2000. "Autonomy and interdependence: Quandaries in genetic decision making." In Mackenzie and Stoljar, pp. 236–58.

Dreger, A. D. 2004. *One of Us: Conjoined Twins and the Future of Normal.* Cambridge, Mass.: Harvard University Press.

Ebbesen, M., and B. D. Pedersen. 2007. "Using empirical research to formulate normative ethical principles in biomedicine." *Medicine, Health Care, and Philosophy* 10:33–48.

Eberly, S. S. 1988. "Fairies and the folklore of disability: Changelings, hybrids and the solitary fairy." *Folklore* 99:58–77.

Edwards, S. D. 2004. "Disability, identity and the 'expressivist objection.'" *Journal of Medical Ethics* 30:418–20.

———. 2005. *Disability: Definitions, Value and Identity*. Abingdon, UK: Radcliffe.

Ells, C. 2001. "Lessons about autonomy from the experience of disability." *Social Theory and Practice* 27:599–615.

Enhanced Surveillance of Meningococcal Disease. National Annual Report: July 2002–June 2003. www.hpa.org.uk/infections/topics_az/meningo/ESMD _annual_ report_0203.pdf. Accessed November 20, 2007.

Fadiman, A. 1998. *The Spirit Catches You and You Fall Down*. New York: Farrar Straus & Giroux.

Fawcett, B. 2000. *Feminist Perspectives on Disability*. New York: Prentice Hall.

Feinberg, J. 1992. "The child's right to an open future." In *Freedom and Fulfillment*, ed. J. Feinberg, pp. 76–97. Princeton, N.J.: Princeton University Press.

Feinstein, A. R. 1975. "Science, clinical medicine and the spectrum of disease." In *Textbook of Medicine*, ed. P. B. Beeson and W. McDermott, pp. 3–6. Philadelphia: Saunders.

Fine, M., and A. Asch. 1988. *Women with Disabilities: Essays in Psychology, Culture, and Politics*. Philadelphia: Temple University Press.

Finger, A. 1990. *Past Due: A Story of Disability, Pregnancy, and Birth*. Seattle: Seal Press.

Fisher, L., and L. Embree, eds. 2000. *Feminist Phenomenology*. Dordrecht: Springer.

Foucault, M. 1991. *Remarks on Marx: Conversations with Duccio Trombadori*. Trans. R. J. Goldstein and J. Cascaito. Brooklyn, N.Y.: Semiotext(e).

Fox, R. C., and J. P. Swazey. 1992. *Spare Parts: Organ Replacement in American Society*. New York: Oxford University Press.

Frank, A. W. 1995. *The Wounded Storyteller: Body, Illness, and Ethics*. Chicago: University of Chicago Press.

Frank, A. W., and T. Jones. 2003. "Bioethics and the later Foucault." *Journal of Medical Humanities* 24:179–86.

Frank, G. 1986. "On embodiment: A case study of congenital limb deficiency in American culture." *Culture, Medicine and Psychiatry* 10:189–219.

———. 2000. *Venus On Wheels: Two Decades of Dialogue on Disability, Biography, and Being Female in America*. Berkeley: University of California Press.

Fraser, N. 2000. "Rethinking recognition." *New Left Review* 3:107–20.

Fraser, N., and A. Honneth. 2003. *Redistribution or Recognition? A Political-Philosophical Exchange*. London: Verso.

Fricker, M. 2006. "Powerlessness and social interpretation." *Episteme* 3:96–108.

———. 2007. *Epistemic Injustice: Power and the Ethics of Knowing*. Oxford: Oxford University Press.

Friedman, M. 1992. "Feminism and Modern Friendship: Dislocating the Community." In *Explorations in Feminist Ethics: Theory and Practice*, ed. E. B. Cole and S. Coultrap-McQuin, pp. 89–100. Bloomington: Indiana University Press.

Fuss, D. 1989. *Essentially Speaking: Feminism, Nature and Difference*. New York: Routledge.

Gadamer, H.-G. 1986. *Truth and Method*. Trans. J. Weinsheimer and D. G. Marshall. New York: Crossroad.

Gallagher, S. 2005. *How the Body Shapes the Mind*. Oxford: Oxford University Press.

Gallagher, S., and J. Cole. 1995. "Body image and body schema in a deafferented subject." *Journal of Mind and Behaviour* 16:369–90.

Gallagher, S., and A. Melzoff. 1996. "The earliest sense of self and others: Merleau-Ponty and recent developmental studies." *Philosophical Psychology* 9:213–36.

Garland-Thomson, R. 2002. "Integrating disability, transforming feminist theory." *NWSA Journal* 14:1–32.

Gergen, K. J. 1991. *The Saturated Self*. New York: Basic Books.

Gerhart, K. A., J. Koziol-McLain, S. R. Lowenstein, and G. G. Whiteneck. 1994. "Quality of life following spinal cord injury: Knowledge and attitudes of emergency care providers." *Annals of Emergency Medicine* 23:807–12.

Gewirth, A. 1988. "Ethical universalism and particularism." *Journal of Philosophy* 85:283–302.

Gibbs, R. W., Jr. 1992. "What do idioms really mean?" *Journal of Memory and Language* 31:485–506.

——. 1996. "Why many concepts are metaphorical." *Cognition* 61:309–19.

——. 2003. "Embodied experience and linguistic meaning." *Brain and Language* 84:1–15.

——. 2005. "Embodiment in metaphorical imagination." In Pecher and Zwaan, pp. 65–92.

Gibbs, R. W., Beitel, D. A., Harrington, M., and P. E. Sanders. 1994. "Taking a stand on the meanings of *stand*: Bodily experiences as motivation for polysemy." *Journal of Semantics* 11:231–51.

Gibbs, R., and H. Colston. 1995. "The cognitive psychological reality of image schemas and their transformations." *Cognitive Linguistics* 6:347–78.

Gibbs, R. W., Jr., P. L. Costa Lima, and E. Francozo. 2004. "Metaphor is grounded in embodied experience." *Journal of Pragmatics* 36:1189–1210.

Gibbs, R., and G. Steen, eds. 1999. *Metaphor in Cognitive Linguistics*. Amsterdam: John Benjamins.

Gilligan, C. 1982. *In a Different Voice: Psychological Theory and Women's Development*. Cambridge, Mass.: Harvard University Press.

Glucksberg, S. 2001. *Understanding Figurative Language*. Oxford: Oxford University Press.

Goffman, E. 1971. *Stigma*. Harmondsworth, UK: Penguin.

Goldenberg, M. J. 2005. "Evidence-based ethics? On evidence-based practice and the 'empirical turn' from normative bioethics." *BMC Medical Ethics* 6:E11. Published online November 8, 2005. doi: 10.1186/1472-6939-6-11.

Goldie, P. 2000. *The Emotions: A Philosophical Exploration*. Oxford: Clarendon.

Greene, J., and J. Haidt. 2002. "How (and where) does moral judgment work?" *Trends in Cognitive Sciences* 6:517–23.

Greene, J. D., R. B. Sommerville, L. E. Nystrom, J. M. Darley, and J. D. Cohen. 2001. "An fMRI investigation of emotional engagement in moral judgment." *Science* 293:2105–8.

Griffiths, M. 1995. *Feminisms and the Self: The Web of Identity*. London: Routledge.

Griffiths, P. E., and E. M. Neumann-Held. 1999. "The many faces of the gene." *BioScience* 49:656–62.

Grosz, E. 1994. *Volatile Bodies: Toward a Corporeal Feminism.* Bloomington: Indiana University Press and Sydney: Allen and Unwin.

———. 1995. *Space, Time and Perversion: Essays on the Politics of Bodies.* New York: Routledge and Sydney: Allen and Unwin.

Gunther, D. F., and D. S. Diekema. 2006. "Attenuating growth in children with profound developmental disability. A new approach to an old dilemma." *Archives of Pediatrics & Adolescent Medicine* 160:1013–17.

Hacking, I. 1986. "Making up people." In *Reconstructing Individualism: Autonomy, Individuality, and the Self in Western Thought,* ed. T. C. Heller and C. Brooke-Rose, pp. 222–36. Stanford, Calif.: Stanford University Press.

Haddon, M. 2003. *The Curious Incident of the Dog in the Night-Time.* London: Random House.

Hafferty, F. W., and S. Foster. 1994. "Decontextualizing disability in the crime mystery genre: The case of the invisible handicap." *Disability and Society* 9:185–206.

Haidt, J. 2001. "The emotional dog and its rational tail: A social intuitionist approach to moral judgment." *Psychological Review* 108:814–34.

Haimes, E. 2002. "What can the social sciences contribute to the study of ethics? Theoretical, empirical and substantive considerations." *Bioethics* 16:89–113.

Haraway, D. J. 1991. "A cyborg manifesto: Science, technology, and socialist-feminism in the late twentieth century." In *Simians, Cyborgs and Women: The Reinvention of Nature,* pp. 149–81. New York: Routledge.

———. 1997. *Modest_Witness@Second_Millennium.FemaleMan©Meets_OncoMouse™: Feminism and Technoscience.* New York: Routledge.

Hardiker, P. 1994. "Thinking and practising otherwise: Disability and child abuse." *Disability and Society* 9:257–63.

Harding, S. 1991. *Whose Science? Whose Knowledge?* Ithaca, N.Y.: Cornell University Press.

———. 1993. Rethinking standpoint epistemology: What is "strong objectivity?" In *Feminist Epistemologies,* ed. L. Alcoff and E. Potter, pp. 49–82. London: Routledge.

———. 1997. "Comment on Hekman's "Truth and method": Feminist standpoint theory revisited: Whose standpoint needs the regimes of truth and reality?" *Signs* 22:382–91.

Harré, R. 1991. *The Singular Self: An Introduction to the Psychology of Personhood.* London: Sage.

Harris, Jennifer. 1995. *The Cultural Meaning of Deafness.* Aldershot: Avebury.

Harris, John. 1995. "Should we attempt to eradicate disability?" *Public Understanding of Science* 4:233–42.

———. 2000. "Is there a coherent self-conception of disability?" *Journal of Medical Ethics* 26:95–100.

———. 2005. "Sex selection and regulated hatred." *Journal of Medical Ethics* 31:291–94.

Hartsock, N. 1987. "The feminist standpoint: Developing the ground for a specifically feminist historical materialism." In *Feminism and Methodology: Social Science Issues,* ed. S. Harding, pp. 157–80. Bloomington: Indiana University Press.

Häyri, M. 2004. "There is a difference between selecting a deaf embryo and deafening a hearing child." *Journal of Medical Ethics* 30:510–12.

Hedgecoe, A. M. 2004. "Critical bioethics: Beyond the social science critique of applied ethics." *Bioethics* 18:120–40.

Hekman, S. J. 1995. *Moral Voices, Moral Selves: Carol Gilligan and Feminist Moral Theory.* University Park: Pennsylvania State University Press.

Helman, C. 1990. *Culture, Health and Illness: An Introduction for Health Professionals.* London: Wright.

Hernandez, B. 2005. "A voice in the chorus: Perspectives of young men of colour on their disabilities, identities, and peer-mentors." *Disability and Society* 20:117–33.

Hevey, D. 1992. *The Creatures Time Forgot: Photography and Disability Imagery.* London: Routledge.

Higgins, P. C. 1980. *Outsiders in a Hearing World: A Sociology of Deafness.* London: Sage.

Hockenberry, J. 1995. *Moving Violations: War Zones, Wheelchairs, and Declarations of Independence.* New York: Hyperion.

Holm, S., and M. Jonas. 2004. *Engaging the World: The Use of Empirical Research in Bioethics and the Regulation of Biotechnology.* Amsterdam: IOS Press.

Holmes, H. B., and L. M. Purdy, eds. 1992. *Feminist Perspectives in Medical Ethics.* Bloomington: Indiana University Press.

Honneth, A. 1996. *The Struggle for Recognition: The Moral Grammar of Social Conflict.* Cambridge, Mass.: MIT Press.

Horgan, O., and M. MacLachlan. 2004. "Psychosocial adjustment to lower limb amputation: A review." *Disability and Rehabilitation* 26:837–50.

Hughes, B. 2002. "Bauman's strangers: Impairment and the invalidation of disabled people in modern and postmodern cultures." *Disability and Society* 17:571–84.

Hume, David [1751]. *An Enquiry Concerning the Principles of Morals.* Sec. 9. Repr. in *Hume's Moral and Political Philosophy,* ed. D. H. Aiken. New York: Hafner, 1968.

Hussain, Y. 2005. "South Asian disabled women: Negotiating identities." *Sociological Review* 53:522–38.

Johnson, H. McB. 2006. *Too Late to Die Young: Nearly True Tales from a Life.* New York: Picador.

Johnson, M. 1987. *The Body in the Mind: The Bodily Basis of Meaning, Imagination, and Reason.* Chicago: University of Chicago Press.

———. 1993. *Moral Imagination: Implications of Cognitive Science for Ethics.* Chicago: University of Chicago Press.

Johnson, R. E., and C. Erting. 1982. "Linguistic socialization in the context of emergent Deaf ethnicity." In *Social Aspects of Deafness,* vol. 1 of *Deaf Children and the Socialization Process,* ed. C. Erting and R. Meisegeier. Washington, D.C.: Gallaudet University Press.

Johnston, T. 2005. "In one's own image: Ethics and the reproduction of deafness." *Journal of Deaf Studies and Deaf Education* 10:426–41.

Jonsen, A. R. 1998. *The Birth of Bioethics.* Oxford: Oxford University Press.

Judson, H. F. 1992. "A history of the science and technology behind gene mapping and sequencing." In Kevles and Hood, pp. 37–82.

Kannapell, B. 1982. "Inside the Deaf community." *Deaf American* 34:23–26.

Kennedy, D. 2003. *Little People: Learning to See the World through My Daughter's Eyes.* New York: Rodale.

Kenny, M. 2004. *The Politics of Identity: Liberal Political Theory and the Dilemmas of Difference*. Cambridge: Polity.

Kerr, A., and T. Shakespeare. 2002. *Genetic Politics: From Eugenics to Genome*. Cheltenham: New Clarion Press.

Kevles, D. J. 1992. "Out of eugenics: The historical politics of the human genome." In Kevles and Hood, pp. 3–36.

Kevles, D. J., and L. Hood, eds. 1992. *The Code of Codes: Scientific and Social Issues in the Human Genome Project*. Cambridge, Mass.: Harvard University Press.

Kisor, H. 1990. *What's That Pig Outdoors?* New York: Hill & Wang.

Kittay, E. F. 1999. *Love's Labor: Essays on Women, Equality, and Dependency*. New York: Routledge.

Kriegel, L. 1987. "The cripple in literature." In *Images of the Disabled, Disabling Images*, ed. A. Gartner and T. Joe, pp. 31–46. New York: Praeger.

Kruks, S. 2001. *Retrieving Experience: Subjectivity and Recognition in Feminist Politics*. Ithaca, N.Y.: Cornell University Press.

Kuhse, H., and P. Singer. 1985. *Should the Baby Live? The Problem of Handicapped Infants*. Oxford: Oxford University Press.

Kymlicka, W. 2002. *Contemporary Political Philosophy: An Introduction*. Oxford: Oxford University Press.

Ladd, P., and M. John. 1991. *Deaf People as a Minority Group: The Political Process. Course D251, Issues in Deafness*. Milton Keynes: Open University Press.

Lakoff, G., and M. Johnson. 1980. *Metaphors We Live By*. Chicago: University of Chicago Press.

———. 1999. *Philosophy in the Flesh*. New York: Basic Books.

———. 2002. "Why cognitive science needs embodied realism." *Cognitive Linguistics* 13:245–63.

Lane, H. 1992. *The Mask of Benevolence: Disabling the Deaf Community*. New York: Alfred Knopf.

Lapper, A. 2005. *My Life in My Hands*. London: Simon & Schuster.

Levy, N. 2002a. "Deafness, culture and choice." *Journal of Medical Ethics* 28:284–85.

———. 2002b. "Reconsidering cochlear implants: The lessons of Martha's Vineyard." *Bioethics* 16:134–53.

Lindemann Nelson, H. 2001. *Damaged Identities, Narrative Repair*. Ithaca, N.Y.: Cornell University Press.

Linton, S. 1998. *Claiming Disability: Knowledge and Identity*. New York: New York University Press.

———. 2005. *My Body Politic*. Ann Arbor: University of Michigan Press.

Little, M. 1996. "Why a feminist approach to bioethics?" *Kennedy Institute of Ethics Journal* 6:1–18.

Lloyd, M. 2005. *Beyond Identity Politics: Feminism, Power and Politics*. London: Sage.

Lovell, T. 2000. "Thinking feminism with and against Bourdieu." *Feminist Theory* 1:11–32.

Lugones, M. 1990. "Playfulness, 'world'-traveling, and loving perception." In *Making Face, Making Soul/Haciendo Caras: Creative and Critical Perspectives by Women of Color*, ed. G. Anzaldua, pp. 390–402. San Francisco: Aunt Lute Foundation.

MacIntyre, A. 1985. *After Virtue: A Study in Moral Theory*. London: Duckworth.

Mackenzie, C., and J. L. Scully. 2007. "Moral imagination, disability and embodiment." *Journal of Applied Philosophy* 24:335–51.

Mackenzie, C., and N. Stoljar, eds. 2000. *Relational Autonomy: Feminist Perspectives on Autonomy, Agency and the Social Self.* New York: Oxford University Press.

Mairs, N. 1996. *Waist-High in the World: A Life Among the Nondisabled.* Boston: Beacon Press.

Major-Kincade, T., J. Tyson, and K. Kennedy. 2001. "Training pediatric house staff in evidence-based ethics: An explanatory controlled trial." *Journal of Perinatology* 21:161–66.

Marks, D. 1999. *Disability: Controversial Debates and Psychosocial Perspectives.* London: Routledge.

McCall, L. 1992. "Does gender fit? Bourdieu, feminism, and conceptions of social order." *Theory and Society* 21:837–67.

Meekosha, H. 1998. "Body battles: Bodies, gender and disability." In Shakespeare, pp. 163–180.

Mehnert, T., H. H. Krauss, R. Nadler, and M. Boyd. 1990. "Correlates of life satisfaction in those with disabling conditions." *Rehabilitation Psychology* 35:3–17.

Merleau-Ponty, M. 1964. *The Primacy of Perception: And Other Essays on Phenomenology, Psychology, the Philosophy of Art, History and Politics,* ed. J. M. Edie. Evanston, Ill.: Northwestern University Press.

———. 1969. *The Visible and the Invisible.* Evanston: Northwestern University Press.

———. [1945] 2002. *The Phenomenology of Perception.* London: Routledge.

Metzger, M., and B. Bahan. 2001. "Discourse Analysis." In *The Sociolinguistics of Sign Languages,* ed. C. Lucas, pp. 112–44. Cambridge University Press.

Meyers, D. T. 1989. *Self, Society, and Personal Choice.* New York: Columbia University Press.

———. 1994. *Subjection and Subjectivity: Psychoanalytic Feminism and Moral Philosophy.* New York: Routledge.

———. 2004. "Narrative and moral life." In *Setting the Moral Compass,* ed. C. Calhoun, pp. 288–305. Oxford: Oxford University Press.

Middleton, A. V., J. V. Hewison, and R. V. Mueller. 1998. "Attitudes of deaf adults towards genetic testing for hereditary deafness." *American Journal of Human Genetics* 63:1175–80.

———. 2001. "Prenatal diagnosis for deafness—what is the potential demand?" *Journal of Genetic Counselling* 10:121–31.

Miller, D. 1992. "Distributive justice: What the people think." *Ethics* 102:555–93.

Moi, T. 1991. "Appropriating Bourdieu: Feminist theory and Pierre Bourdieu's sociology of culture." *New Literary History* 22:1017–49.

Molewijk, B., A. M. Stiggelbout, W. Otten, H. M. Dupuis, and J. Kievit. 2004. "Empirical data and moral theory. A plea for integrated empirical ethics." *Medicine, Health Care, and Philosophy* 7:55–69.

Moll, J., R. de Oliveira-Souza, P. J. Eslinger, I. E. Bramati, J. Mourão-Miranda, P. A. Andreiuolo, and L. Pessoa. 2002. "The neural correlates of moral sensitivity: A functional magnetic resonance imaging investigation of basic and moral emotions." *Journal of Neuroscience* 22:2730–36.

Morris, J. 1991. *Pride against Prejudice: Transforming Attitudes to Disability.* London: Women's Press.

Morrow, A. 2004. "Identity politics and disability studies: A critique of recent theory." *Michigan Quarterly Review* 43:269–96.

Mundy, L. 2002. "A world of their own." *Washington Post Magazine*, March 31.

Murphy, G. L. 1996. "On metaphorical representation." *Cognition* 60:173–204.

Murphy, R. 1987. *The Body Silent*. New York: Henry Holt.

Musschenga, A. W. 1999. "Empirical science and ethical theory: The case of informed consent." In *Reasoning in Ethics and Law: The Role of Theory, Principles and Facts*, ed. A. W. Musschenga and W. van der Steen, pp. 183–205. Aldershot: Ashgate.

Nagel, T. 1989. *The View from Nowhere*. Oxford: Oxford University Press.

Nedelsky, J. 1989. "Reconceiving autonomy: Sources, thoughts and possibilities." *Yale Journal of Law and Feminism* 1:7–36.

Nelson, J. L. 2000a. "Prenatal diagnosis, personal identity, and disability." *Kennedy Institute of Ethics Journal* 10:213–28.

———. 2000b. "Moral teachings from unexpected quarters: Lessons for bioethics from the social sciences and managed care." *Hastings Center Report* 32:12–17.

———. 2001. "Knowledge, authority and identity: A prolegomenon to an epistemology of the clinic." *Theoretical Medicine* 22:107–22.

Neumann-Held, E., and C. Rehmann-Sutter, eds. 2006. *Genes in Development: Rereading the Molecular Paradigm*. Durham, N.C. and London: Duke University Press.

Nikku N., and B. E. Eriksson. 2006. "Microethics in action." *Bioethics* 20:169–79.

Noddings, N. 1984. *Caring: A Feminine Approach to Ethics and Moral Education*. Berkeley: University of California Press.

Norden, M. 1995. *The Cinema of Isolation*. New Brunswick, N.J.: Rutgers University Press.

Nussbaum, M. C. 1995. "Human capabilities, female human beings." In *Women, Culture and Development: A Study of Human Capabilities*, ed. M. C. Nussbaum and J. Glover, pp. 61–104. New York: Oxford University Press.

Oakley, A. 1981. "Interviewing women: A contradiction in terms." In *Doing Feminist Research*, ed. Helen Roberts, pp. 30–61. New York: Routledge.

Oliver, M. 1990. *The Politics of Disablement*. Basingstoke, UK: Macmillan.

———. 1996. *Understanding Disability: From Theory to Practice*. Basingstoke, UK: Macmillan.

Olney, M. F., and K. F. Brockelman. 2003. "Out of the disability closet: Strategic use of perception management by select university students with disabilities." *Disability and Society* 18:35–50.

Oyama, S., P. E. Griffiths, and R. D. Gray, eds. 2003. *Cycles of Contingency: Developmental Systems and Evolution*. Cambridge, Mass.: MIT Press.

Padden, C., and T. Humphries. 1994. *Deaf in America: Voices from a Culture*. Cambridge, Mass.: Harvard University Press.

———. 2005. *Inside Deaf Culture*. Cambridge, Mass.: Harvard University Press.

Pallasch, A. M. 2007. "Denied service for using her feet, woman claims." *Chicago Sun-Times*, July 2.

Parens, E. 2006. *Surgically Shaping Children: Technology, Ethics, and the Pursuit of Normality*. Baltimore: Johns Hopkins University Press.

Parens, E., and A. Asch. 2002. *Prenatal Testing and Disability Rights*. Washington, D.C.: Georgetown University Press.

Parker, M. 2007. "The best possible child." *Journal of Medical Ethics* 33:279–83.

Pecher, D., and R. A. Zwaan, eds. 2005. *Grounding Cognition: The Role of Perception and Action in Memory, Language, and Thinking.* Cambridge: Cambridge University Press.

Pellegrino, E. 1995. "The limitation of empirical research in ethics." *Journal of Clinical Ethics* 6:161–62.

Peters, S. 2000. "Is there a disability culture? A syncretisation of three possible world views." *Disability and Society* 15:583–601.

Phillips, A. 1998. *The Beast in the Nursery.* London: Faber and Faber.

Preston, P. 2001. *Mother Father Deaf: Living between Sound and Silence.* Cambridge, Mass.: Harvard University Press.

Price, J., and M. Shildrick. 1998. "Uncertain thoughts on the dis/abled body." In *Vital Signs: Feminist Reconfigurations of the Bio/logical Body,* ed. M. Shildrick and J. Price, pp. 224–49. Edinburgh: Edinburgh University Press.

Prinz, J. J. 2005. "Passionate thoughts: The emotional embodiment of moral concepts." In Pecher and Zwaan, pp. 93–114.

Rabinow, P., and N. Rose. 2006. "Biopower today." *Biosocieties* 1:195–217.

Rapp, R. 2000. *Testing Women, Testing the Fetus: The Social Impact of Amniocentesis in America.* New York: Routledge.

Rawlinson, M. C. 2001. "The concept of a feminist bioethics." *Journal of Medicine and Philosophy* 26:405–16.

Rawls, J. A. 1971. *A Theory of Justice.* Oxford: Oxford University Press.

Rée, J. 1999. *I See a Voice: Language, Deafness and the Senses—a Philosophical History.* London: HarperCollins.

Reeve, D. 2002. "Negotiating psycho-emotional dimensions of disability and their influence on identity constructions." *Disability and Society* 17:493–508.

Rehmann-Sutter, C. 1999. "Contextual bioethics." *Perspektiven der Philosophie* 25:315–38.

———. 2002. "Genetics, embodiment and identity." In *On Human Nature: Anthropological, Biological, and Philosophical Foundations,* ed. A. Grunwald, M. Gutmann, and E. M. Neumann-Held, pp. 23–50. Berlin: Springer.

Rehmann-Sutter, C., Düwell, M., and D. Mieth, eds. 2006. *Bioethics in Cultural Contexts: Reflections on Methods and Finitude.* Dordrecht: Springer.

Reindal, S. M. 1999. "Independence, dependence, interdependence: Some reflections on the subject of personal autonomy." *Disability and Society* 14:353–67.

Richardson, D. C., M. J. Spivey, L. W. Barsalou, and K. McRae. 2003. "Spatial representations activated during real-time comprehension of verbs." *Cognitive Science* 27:767–80.

Riis, J., G. Loewenstein, J. Baron, C. Jepson, A. Fagerlin, and P. A. Ubel. 2005. "Ignorance of hedonic adaptation to hemodialysis: A study using ecological momentary assessment." *Journal of Experimental Psychology* 134:3–9.

Riley, R. 2002. "Pair seeks IVF deaf gene test." *Herald Sun,* June 30.

Rose, J. 1983. "Femininity and its discontents." *Feminist Review* 14:5–21.

Ross, K. 1997. "But where's me in it? Disability, broadcasting and the audience." *Media, Culture & Society* 19:669–77.

Rothman, D. J. 1991. *Strangers at the Bedside: A History of How Law and Bioethics Transformed Medical Decision Making.* New York: Basic Books.

Rozin, P., L. Lowery, S. Imada, and J. Haidt. 1999. "The CAD triad hypothesis: A mapping between three moral emotions (contempt, anger, disgust) and three moral codes (community, autonomy, divinity)." *Journal of Personality and Social Psychology* 76:574–86.

Ryan, D. T., and J. S. Schuchman, eds. 2002. *Deaf People in Hitler's Europe*. Washington, D.C.: Gallaudet University Press.

Sacks, O. 1989. *Seeing Voices: A Journey into the World of the Deaf*. Berkeley: University of California Press.

Sallis, J. 1981. *Merleau-Ponty: Perception, Structure, Language*. Atlantic Highlands, N.J.: Humanities Press.

Savulescu, J. 2001. "Procreative beneficence: Why we should select the best children." *Bioethics* 15:413–26.

———. 2002. "Deaf lesbians, 'designer disability,' and the future of medicine." *British Medical Journal* 325:771–73.

———. 2007. "In defence of procreative beneficence." *Journal of Medical Ethics* 33:284–88.

Schachter, D. L. 2001. *The Seven Sins of Memory: How the Mind Forgets and Remembers*. New York: Houghton Mifflin.

Schmidt, E. B. 2007. "The parental obligation to expand a child's range of open futures when making genetic trait selections for their child." *Bioethics* 21:191–97.

Scott, J. W. 1991. "The evidence of experience." *Critical Enquiry* 17:773–97.

Scully, J. L. 2002. "A postmodern disorder: Moral encounters with molecular models of disability." In *Disability/Postmodernity: Embodying Disability Theory*, ed. M. Corker and T. Shakespeare, pp. 48–61. London: Continuum.

———. 2006a. "Nothing like a gene." In Neumann-Held and Rehmann-Sutter, pp. 349–64.

———. 2006b. "Disabled embodiment and an ethic of care." In Rehmann-Sutter et al., pp. 247–61.

Scully, J. L., R. Porz, and C. Rehmann-Sutter. 2007. "You don't make genetic test decisions from one day to the next. Using time to preserve moral space." *Bioethics* 21:208–17.

Scully, J. L., and C. Rehmann-Sutter. 2001. "When norms normalize: The case of genetic enhancement." *Human Gene Therapy* 12:87–96.

Scully, J. L., C. Rippberger, and C. Rehmann-Sutter. 2004. "Non-professionals' evaluations of gene therapy ethics." *Social Science & Medicine* 58:1415–25.

Shakespeare, T., ed. 1998. *The Disability Reader: Social Science Perspectives*. London: Cassell.

Shakespeare, T. 2006. *Disability Rights and Wrongs*. Abingdon, UK: Routledge.

Shakespeare, T., K. Gillespie-Sells, and D. Davies. 1996. *The Sexual Politics of Disability*. London: Cassell.

Shakespeare, T., and N. Watson. 1996. "The body line controversy. A new direction in disability studies?" Available online from the Disability Archive, Leeds University: www.leeds.ac.uk/disabilitystudies/archiveuk/Shakespeare/The%20body%20line%20controversy.pdf.

———. 2001. "The social model of disability: An outdated ideology?" *Exploring Theories and Expanding Methodologies: Research in Social Science and Disability* 2:9–28.

Sherwin, S. 1992. *No Longer Patient: Feminist Ethics and Health Care.* Philadelphia: Temple University Press.

Sherwin, S., F. Baylis, M. Bell, M. De Koninck, J. Downie, A. Lippmann, M. Lock, W. Mitchinson, K. Pauly Morgan, J. Mosher, and B. Parish, eds. 1998. *The Politics of Women's Health.* Philadelphia: Temple University Press.

Shildrick, M. 1997. *Leaky Bodies and Boundaries: Feminism, Postmodernism and (Bio)ethics.* London: Routledge.

Shildrick, M., and R. Mykitiuk, eds. 2005. *Ethics of the Body: Postconventional Challenges.* Cambridge, Mass.: MIT Press.

Shusterman, R. 2005. "The silent, limping body of philosophy." In *The Cambridge Companion to Merleau-Ponty,* ed. T. Carman and M. Hansen, pp. 151–80. Cambridge: Cambridge University Press.

Shweder, R. A., N. C. Much, M. Mahapatra, and L. Park. 1997. "The 'big three' of morality (autonomy, community, divinity), and the 'big three' explanations of suffering." In *Morality and Health,* ed. A. Brandt and P. Rozin, pp. 119–69. New York: Routledge.

Siebers, T. 2005. "Disability as masquerade." In *Difference and Identity: A Special Issue of Literature and Medicine,* ed. J. M. Metzl and S. Poirier, pp. 1–22. Baltimore, Md.: Johns Hopkins University Press.

Silvers, A. 1995. "Reconciling equality to difference: Caring (f)or justice for people with disabilities." *Hypatia* 10:30–55.

———. 2005. "Predicting genetic disability while commodifying health." In Wasserman et al., pp. 43–66.

Singleton, J. L., and M. D. Tittle. 2000. "Deaf parents and their hearing children." *Journal of Deaf Studies and Deaf Education* 5:221–36.

Smith, D. 1990. *The Conceptual Practices of Power: A Feminist Sociology of Knowledge.* Boston: Northeastern University Press.

Smolens, J. 1996. "An interview with André Dubus." *AWP Chronicle* 29:1–6.

Solomon, A. 1994. "Defiantly deaf." *New York Times Magazine,* August 28. At query.nytimes.com/gst/fullpage.html?res=9A00E2D91639F93BA1575BC0A9629 58260&sec=&spon=&pagewanted=10. Accessed November 19, 2007.

Somers, M. R. 1994. "The narrative constitution of identity: A relational and network approach." *Theory and Society* 23:605–49.

Sparrow, R. 2005. "Defending Deaf culture: The case of cochlear implants." *Journal of Political Philosophy* 13:135–52.

Spivak, G. 1990a. Interview with Elizabeth Grosz. Repr. as "Criticism, feminism and the institution." In *The Post-Colonial Critic: Interviews, Strategies, Dialogues,* ed. S. Harasym, pp. 1–16. New York: Routledge.

———. 1990b. "Practical politics of the open end." In *The Post-Colonial Critic: Interviews, Strategies, Dialogues,* ed. S. Harasym, pp. 95–112. New York: Routledge.

Stemp, J. 2004. "Devices and desires: Science fiction, fantasy and disability in literature for young people." *Disability Studies Quarterly* 24. At www.dsq-sds -archives.org/_articles_html/2004/winter/dsq_w04_stemp.html. Accessed June 18, 2008.

Stensman, R. 1985. "Severely mobility disabled people assess the quality of their lives." *Scandinavian Journal of Rehabilitative Medicine* 17:87–99.

Stern, S. J., K. S. Arnos, L. Murrelle, K. O. Welch, W. E. Nance, and A. Pandya. 2002. "Attitudes of deaf and hard of hearing subjects towards genetic testing and prenatal diagnosis of hearing loss." *Journal of Medical Genetics* 39:449–53.

Stiggelbout, A., B. Molewijk, W. Otten, D. Timmermans, H. VanBockel, and J. Kievit. 2004. "Ideals of patient autonomy in clinical decision-making: A study on the development of a scale to access patients' and physicians' views." *Journal of Medical Ethics* 30:268–74.

Stoetzler M., and N. Yuval-Davis. 2002. "Standpoint theory, situated knowledge and the situated imagination." *Feminist Theory* 3:315–33.

Sugarman, J. 2004. "The future of empirical research in bioethics." *Journal of Law and Medical Ethics* 32:226–31.

Taylor, C. 1994. The Politics of Recognition. In *Multiculturalism*, ed. A. Gutman, pp. 22–73. Princeton, N.J.: Princeton University Press.

———. 2004. "An End to Mediational Epistemology." Lecture given at Trinity College, University of Toronto, November 11. At goodreads.ca/lectures/taylor/larkin-stuart04.html. Accessed September 1, 2007.

Thelen, E. 1995. "Motor development: A new synthesis." *American Psychologist* 50:79–95.

Thelen, E., and L Smith. 1994. *A Dynamic Systems Approach to the Development of Cognition and Action*. Cambridge: MIT Press.

Thomas, C. 2007. *Sociologies of Disability and Illness*. Basingstoke, UK: Palgrave Macmillan.

Tong, R., A. Donchin, and S. Dodds, eds. 2004. *Linking Visions: Feminist Bioethics, Human Rights, and the Developing World*. Lanham, Md: Rowman & Littlefield.

Toombs, K. 1993. *The Meaning of Illness: A Phenomenological Account of the Different Perspectives of Physician and Patient*. Dordrecht: Kluwer.

Tremain, S., ed. 2005. *Foucault and the Government of Disability*. Ann Arbor: University of Michigan Press.

Tronto, J. 1993. *Moral Boundaries: A Political Argument for an Ethic of Care*. New York: Routledge.

Turner, L. 2004. "Bioethics in pluralistic societies." *Medicine, Health Care and Philosophy* 7:201–8.

Tyson, J. E., and B. J. Stoll. 2003. "Evidence-based ethics and the care and outcome of extremely premature infants." *Clinics in Perinatology* 30:363–87.

Ubel, P. A., G. Loewenstein, N. Schwarz, and D. Smith. 2005. "Misimagining the unimaginable: The disability paradox and health care decision making." *Health Psychology* 24 suppl. S:57–62.

UPIAS. 1976. *Fundamental Principles of Disability*. London: UPIAS.

van der Scheer, L., and G. Widdershoven. 2004. "Integrated empirical ethics: Loss of normativity?" *Medicine, Health Care and Philosophy* 7:71–9.

van Rompay, T., P. Hekkert, D. Saakes, and B. Russo. 2005. "Grounding abstract object characteristics in embodied interactions." *Acta Psychologica (Amsterdam)* 119:315–51.

Vehmas, S. 2003. "Live and let die? Disability in bioethics." *New Review of Bioethics* 1:145–57.

Ville, I., M. Crost, J.-F. Ravaud, and Tetrafig Group. 2003. "Disability and a sense of community belonging. A study among tetraplegic spinal-cord-injured persons in France." *Social Science & Medicine* 56:321–32.

Ville, I., and J.-F. Ravaud. 2001. "Subjective well-being and severe motor impairments. The Tetrafig survey on the long-term outcome of tetraplegic spinal cord injured persons." *Social Science & Medicine* 52:369–84.

Wade, C. M. 1994. "Identity." *Disability Rag and ReSource* 16:32–36.

Walker, L. A. 1986. *A Loss for Words: The Story of Deafness in a Family*. New York: Harper & Row.

Walker, M. U. 1998. *Moral Understandings: A Feminist Study in Ethics*. New York: Routledge.

———. 2002. "Morality in practice: A response to Claudia Card and Lorraine Code." *Hypatia* 17:174–82.

———. 2003. *Moral Contexts*. Lanham, Md.: Rowman & Littlefield.

Wasserman, D., J. Bickerbach, and R. Wachbroit, eds. 2005. *Quality of Life and Human Difference: Genetic Testing, Health Care, and Disability*. New York: Cambridge University Press.

Watson, J. D., and R. M. Cook-Deegan. 1991. "Origins of the Human Genome Project." *FASEB Journal* 5:8–11.

Watson, N. 2002. "Well, I know this is going to sound very strange to you, but I don't see myself as a disabled person: Identity and disability." *Disability and Society* 17:509–27.

Webb, J., T. Schirato, and G. Danaher. 2002. *Understanding Bourdieu*. London: Sage.

Weiss, G. 1999. *Body Images: Embodiment as Intercorporeality*. New York: Routledge.

Wendell, S. 1996. *The Rejected Body: Feminist Philosophical Reflections on Disability*. New York: Routledge.

West, P. 1969. *Words for a Deaf Daughter*. London: Gollancz.

Westermann, G., S. Sirois, T. R. Shultz, and D. Mareschal. 2006. "Modelling developmental cognitive neuroscience." *Trends in Cognitive Sciences* 10:227–32.

Whitebrook, M. 2001. *Identity, Narrative and Politics*. London: Routledge.

Whitney, C. 2006. "Intersections in identity—identity development among queer women with disabilities." *Sexuality and Disability* 24:39–52.

Widdershoven, G. A. M. 1993. "The story of life. Hermeneutic perspectives on the relationship between narrative and life history." In *The Narrative Study of Lives*, ed. R. Josselson and A. Lieblich, vol. 1, pp. 1–29. Newbury Park, Calif.: Sage.

Wilfond, B. S. 2007. "The Ashley case: The public response and policy implications." *Hastings Center Report* 37:12–13.

Williams, G. 2001. "Theorizing disability." In *The Disability Studies Handbook*, ed. G. Albrecht, K. Seelman, and M. Bury, pp. 123–44. London: Sage.

Wilson, M. 2002. "Six views of embodied cognition." *Psychonomic Bulletin & Review* 9:625–36.

World Health Organization. 1980. *International Classification of Impairments, Disabilities and Handicaps*. Geneva: World Health Organization.

———. 2001. *International Classification of Functioning, Disability and Health*. Geneva: World Health Organization.

Young, I. M. 1990. *Justice and the Politics of Difference*. Princeton, N.J.: Princeton University Press.

———. 2000. *Inclusion and Democracy*. Oxford: Oxford University Press.

———. 2005. *On Female Body Experience: "Throwing like a Girl" and Other Essays*. Oxford: Oxford University Press.

Zussman, R. 2000. "The contributions of sociology to medical ethics." *Hastings Center Report* 30:7–11.

Index

abuse, sexual and physical, 50, 99, 170
achondroplasia, 62, 110
agency, moral, 34, 35, 46, 66, 102, 109,
  112, 113, 114, 115, 116, 127, 128,
  129, 130, 133, 134, 136, 144, 145,
  148, 150, 160, 161, 162, 167. *See
  also* moral agent
anxiety caused by disability, 114,
  117–18
Appiah, Kwame Anthony, 115, 138,
  141–42
Asch, Adrienne, 141
automythology, 120–22
autonomy, 3, 62, 63, 75, 91 99, 101–2,
  160–63, 166–68, 177n; relational,
  161–62, 167. *See also* self-
  determination

being-in-the-world, 84–87, 94, 104nn
beneficence, 160
Berkeley Center for Independent
  Living, 122
biological/genetic reductionism, 5–7,
  24
biopower, 36, 157
blind, 20, 22, 96, 117, 127. *See also*
  visual impairment
Blunkett, David, 20, 37n

body image, 13, 88, 104n
body schema, 87–89, 94–97, 103,
  104nn, 167–68
Bourdieu, Pierre, 13, 64–69, 71, 79, 80,
  83–84, 99; feminist critique of
  67–68. *See also* habitus
brain-machine interface, 96
Brentano, Franz Clemens, 84
Butler, Judith, 28

Calhoun, Cheshire, 148
care, 76–78, 160. *See also* dependence;
  independence
care ethics, 164–66
carers, 43, 48, 116, 118, 158, 165, 167
central disability paradox, 63–64
Chorost, Michael, 78, 127–28, 133
cochlear implant(ation), 10, 48, 77, 78,
  81n, 127–28, 157
cognition, higher-order, 84, 85, 87, 89,
  90, 91, 92, 93, 97, 167
cognitive impairments. *See* learning
  disability
cognitive science, 13, 14, 64, 85,
  89–93, 95, 97, 100, 103, 104n, 167
  See also neuroscience
community, 46, 48, 63–64, 73–75,
  77–78, 81n, 128, 129, 174; found,

About the Author

Jackie Leach Scully is senior lecturer at the School of Geography, Politics and Sociology, and a member of the Policy, Ethics and Life Sciences Research Centre, Newcastle University, UK. She took her first degree in biochemistry at the University of Oxford and her Ph.D. in molecular biology at the University of Cambridge, followed by research fellowships at the Swiss Cancer Research Institute in Epalinges and the Institute of Physiology, University of Basel. After work in public engagement and medical education she joined the Unit for Ethics in the Biosciences in Basel in 1997, moving to Newcastle in 2006. She has held visiting fellowships at Macquarie University, New South Wales, and at the ECAV Academy of the Arts, Valais, Switzerland, and is honorary senior lecturer in the Faculty of Medicine, University of Sydney. Jackie Leach Scully has been active in the disability movement in Britain and Europe since the early 1980s. Her main research interests are in moral understandings of novel biomedical technologies, disability and embodiment, religion and bioethics, and feminist and psychoanalytic approaches. Her work has been published in *Bioethics, Social Science and Medicine, New Genetics and Society, Sociology of Health and Illness,* and the *Journal of Applied Philosophy;* she is the author of *Quaker Approaches to Moral Issues in Genetics* (2002) and coedited *Good and Evil: Quaker Perspectives* (2007) and *Gekauftes Gewissen? Zur Rolle der Bioethik in Institutionen* (2007).